PREFACE

Often as a nursing student and even as a practicing nurse, you will face challenging client situations that test your knowledge base, your ability to prioritize, and your familiarity with certain skills. The *Clinical Handbook for Contemporary Maternal-Newborn Nursing* has been created to help you in situations like these. The handbook provides succinct, pertinent information about the antepartum, intrapartum, newborn, and postpartum client. Each content area includes key information about medical therapy as well as nursing care information organized according to the nursing process. Critical nursing assessments and interventions are identified, and specific suggestions are given regarding documentation of care.

In addition to serving as a resource for normal childbearing, as well as selected complications, the handbook includes practical features to assist the nurse. Procedures specific to the maternal-child clinical area are included to help you provide nursing care. Commonly used medications are presented in the Drug Guide section. A specifically developed appendix with Spanish translations of some key phrases used in the maternal-child area is designed to assist the nurse who does not speak Spanish. Another appendix contains information about working with deaf clients through an interpreter.

Although the handbook gives condensed information about each subject area, critical aspects of nursing practice have been included. It is our hope that this book will enhance maternal-newborn nursing practice and help nurses provide safe, competent care to all mothers and babies.

We would like to express our appreciation to the Pearson Health Science team for their encouragement, support, and assistance with this project. Kim Mortimer, our editor, is a constant source of support and encouragement. We are also grateful to editorial assistant Sarah Wrocklage and production editor Anne Garcia. Thanks, too, to Erin Melloy, project editor at S4Carlisle Publishing Services.

Finally, we would like to express our heartfelt appreciation to our nursing students, who brighten each day. By being with them, we gain an understanding of their struggle to master an ever-growing body of knowledge. We have incorporated many of their requests and ideas into the information that appears in this handbook. As always, it is our goal to provide a tool that students and practicing nurses will find helpful.

PWL
MLL
MRD

Clinical Handbook for
CONTEMPORARY MATERNAL-NEWBORN NURSING CARE

SEVENTH EDITION

Clinical Handbook for
CONTEMPORARY MATERNAL-NEWBORN NURSING CARE

SEVENTH EDITION

Patricia A. Wieland Ladewig, PhD, RN

Marcia L. London, RNC, MSN, APRN, CNS, NNP-BC

Michele R. Davidson, PhD, CNM, CFN, RN

Pearson

Boston   Columbus   Indianapolis   New York
San Francisco   Upper Saddle River   Amsterdam
Cape Town   Dubai   London   Madrid   Milan   Munich
Paris   Montreal   Toronto   Delhi   Mexico City   Sao Paulo
Sydney   Hong Kong   Seoul   Singapore   Taipei   Tokyo

Library of Congress Cataloging-in-Publication Data

London, Marcia L.
Clinical handbook for contemporary maternal-newborn nursing care/Marcia L. London,
Patricia A. Wieland Ladewig. –7th ed.
    p. ; cm.
Includes bibliographical references and index.
ISBN-10: 0-13-504725-0
ISBN-13: 978-0-13-504725-5
1. Maternity nursing–Handbooks, manuals, etc. I. Ladewig, Patricia W. II. Title.
[DNLM: 1. Maternal–Child Nursing–Handbooks. WY 49 L847c 2010]
RG951.O4327 2010
618.2'0231–dc22
                    2009014845

Notice: Care has been taken to confirm the accuracy of information presented in this
book. The authors, editors, and the publisher, however, cannot accept any responsibility
for errors or omissions or for consequences from application of the information in this
book and make no warranty, express or implied, with respect to its contents.
    The authors and publisher have exerted every effort to ensure that drug selections
and dosages set forth in this text are in accord with current recommendations and practice
at time of publication. However, in view of ongoing research, changes in government
regulations, and the constant flow of information relating to drug therapy and reactions,
the reader is urged to check the package inserts of all drugs for any change in indications
or dosage and for added warning and precautions. This is particularly important when the
recommended agent is a new and/or infrequently employed drug.

Pearson Education Ltd., London
Pearson Education Singapore, Pte. Ltd
Pearson Education Canada, Inc.
Pearson Education—Japan
Pearson Education Australia PTY, Limited

Pearson Education North Asia, Ltd., Hong Kong
Pearson Educación de Mexico, S.A. de C.V.
Pearson Education Malaysia, Pte. Ltd.
Pearson Education Upper Saddle River, New Jersey

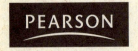

10 9 8 7 6 5 4 3 2 1
ISBN-13: 978-013504725-5
ISBN-10: 0-13-504725-0

CONTENTS

1 THE ANTEPARTAL CLIENT

During the antepartal period, nursing interventions focus primarily on client teaching and ongoing monitoring of the woman so that any potential complications are detected promptly. Teaching typically focuses on nutrition, on interventions to deal with the common discomforts of pregnancy, and on self-care activities indicated throughout pregnancy.

PREGNANCY LENGTH
- Due date (date on which the baby is expected) is calculated from the first day of a woman's last menstrual period (LMP). (See page 15 for description of calculation.)
- Pregnancy lasts about 9 calendar months, 10 lunar months, 40 weeks, or 280 days.
- Conception actually occurs about 14 days before the start of a woman's next menstrual period. Thus, the actual time she is pregnant is about 2 weeks less, or 266 days.

Trimesters
- Pregnancy is considered in terms of trimesters, which each last three calendar months.
- First trimester: The woman usually learns she is pregnant and may seek prenatal care. The first trimester is the time of primary organ development for the fetus.
- Second trimester: Many consider this the most tranquil time for the pregnant woman. Morning sickness passes, and quickening (feeling the baby move) occurs.
- Third trimester: The woman becomes anxious for the pregnancy to end. She may feel awkward because of

her increasing weight and the physical and psychologic changes she experiences.

NORMAL PHYSICAL CHANGES OF PREGNANCY

Uterus

- Uterus increases dramatically in size and weight.
- *Braxton Hicks contractions* begin by the end of the first trimester. These are rhythmic contractions of the uterus that are painless initially but become noticeable, and sometimes uncomfortable, toward term (the end of pregnancy). They are then referred to as "false labor." Braxton Hicks contractions are palpable during bimanual exam by the fourth month and palpable abdominally by the 28th week.

Cervix

- Glandular tissue increases in number and becomes hyperactive.
- Mucous plug is formed in cervix and acts as a barrier to prevent ascending infection.
- Increased blood flow to cervix leads to softening (*Goodell's sign*) and bluish coloration (*Chadwick's sign*). Goodell's sign and Chadwick's sign are visible on speculum examination.

Ovaries

- Ovum production ceases. Corpus luteum persists and secretes hormones until weeks 6–8.

Vagina

- Increased vascularity produces bluish color (Chadwick's sign).
- Epithelium hypertrophies.

Breasts

- Size and nodularity increase; some increased tenderness occurs.

- Superficial veins are prominent.
- Increased pigmentation of areola and nipples occurs.
- *Colostrum* is usually produced by week 12. (Colostrum is the antibody-rich forerunner of mature breast milk.) Women who are not visibly secreting colostrum need reassurance that they are producing it even if it is not evident.

Respiratory System

- Some hyperventilation occurs as pregnancy progresses.
- Tidal volume increases; airway resistance decreases.
- Diaphragm is elevated; substernal angle is increased.
- Breathing changes from abdominal to thoracic.

Cardiovascular System

- Blood volume increases about 40%–45%.
- Systemic and pulmonary vascular resistance decreases.
- Cardiac output increases 30%–50% over prepregnant levels, peaks at 25–30 weeks' gestation, and generally remains elevated for duration of pregnancy.
- Pulse rate increases.
- Blood pressure (BP) decreases slightly by second trimester and is near prepregnant levels at term.
- Pressure of enlarging uterus on vena cava can interfere with blood return to the heart and cause dizziness, pallor, clamminess, and lowered BP. This condition is called *supine hypotensive syndrome* or *vena caval syndrome*. It may also be called *aortocaval compression* because the uterus may exert pressure on the aorta and its collateral circulation. The condition is corrected by having the woman lie on her side or lie with a wedge under her right hip.
- Red blood cells and hemoglobin levels increase, as does the plasma level. Because plasma volume increases more, a physiologic anemia of pregnancy results, evident in an apparent decrease in hematocrit (Hct). Hct levels of 32%–44% are considered normal.

- Leukocyte production increases to levels of 5,600–12,200/mm^3. Levels may reach 20,000–30,000/mm^3 during labor.
- Fibrin, fibrinogen, and factors VII, VIII, IX, and X increase.

Gastrointestinal System
- Nausea is common; vomiting occurs occasionally.
- *Ptyalism* (excessive salivation) is an occasional problem.
- Intestines and stomach are displaced by uterus.
- Relaxed cardiac sphincter leads to reflux of acidic secretions, resulting in heartburn.
- Delayed gastric emptying leads to constipation.
- Hemorrhoids may develop.

Urinary Tract
- Increased pressure on the bladder from the growing uterus during the first and third trimesters leads to urinary frequency.
- Glomerular filtration rate and renal plasma flow increase.
- Incidence of glycosuria increases, which may be normal or may indicate gestational diabetes mellitus (see Chapter 2).

Skin and Hair
- Pigmentation of areola, nipples, vulva, and linea nigra increases.
- Facial *chloasma* or *melasma gravidarum*, a butterfly-shaped area of pigmentation over the face, may develop. Called the "mask of pregnancy," it usually fades after childbirth.
- *Striae*, or stretch marks, may develop on the abdomen, breasts, and thighs.
- *Vascular spider nevi*, small, bright-red elevations of the skin radiating from the central body, may develop.
- Rate of hair growth may decrease.

Musculoskeletal System

- Joints of pelvis relax somewhat.
- Waddling gait develops because of changed center of gravity and accentuated lumbosacral curve.
- Separation of rectus abdominis muscle, called *diastasis recti*, may occur.

SIGNS OF PREGNANCY

Subjective (Presumptive) Changes

- Symptoms are experienced by the woman.
- Conditions other than pregnancy may be the cause.
- Signs include the following: amenorrhea, nausea and vomiting, excessive fatigue, urinary frequency, changes in the breasts, and *quickening* (mother's perception of fetal movement).

Objective (Probable) Changes

- Signs are perceived by the examiner.
- Conditions other than pregnancy may be the cause.
- Signs include the following: changes in the pelvic organs such as Goodell's sign, Chadwick's sign, and *Hegar's sign* (softening of the isthmus, the area between the cervix and the body of the uterus); enlargement of the abdomen; Braxton Hicks contractions; *uterine souffle* (soft blowing sound heard when auscultating the abdomen, caused by blood pulsating through the placenta); changes in pigmentation of the skin (chloasma [melasma], linea nigra); abdominal striae; fetal outline palpable during examination; and positive pregnancy test.

Diagnostic (Positive) Changes

- Signs are completely objective and caused only by pregnancy.
- Signs include the following: verification of a gestational sac or fetal parts and heartbeat through ultrasonography, as well as detection of fetal heartbeat and fetal movements by a trained examiner.

PSYCHOLOGIC RESPONSES OF THE MOTHER TO PREGNANCY

Unless the following responses are extreme or exaggerated, they are considered normal. They are related to hormonal changes and to the body's efforts to prepare for childbirth and parenting.

Ambivalence

- Ambivalence is common initially, even if pregnancy is planned.
- Mother may have concerns about her career, her relationship with her partner, financial implications, and role change.
- She may make comments such as, "I thought I wanted a baby, but now I'm not so sure."

Acceptance of Pregnancy

- As acceptance grows, the woman shows a high degree of tolerance for the discomforts she may experience in the first trimester.
- In the second trimester, she begins to wear maternity clothes.
- She begins to perceive movement at about 17–20 weeks. She may make comments such as, "Feeling the baby move makes it all seem real" or "It's finally sinking in that I'm going to be a mother."

Introversion

- The expectant woman typically becomes more inwardly focused, less interested in outside activities.
- She is using this time to plan and adjust.
- Her partner may see this as excluding him. She may say, "I never used to like to be alone, but now I like having time to myself just to think and plan."

Mood Swings

- Mood swings from joy to sadness are common and difficult for the woman and her family.

- The woman often feels a great need for love and affection, but her partner, confused by her emotional changes, may react by withdrawing. She may say, "I'm not usually so emotional, but lately any little thing can set me off."

Changes in Body Image

- The woman tends to feel somewhat negative about her body as pregnancy progresses.
- Her increasing abdomen coupled with the waddling gait of pregnancy may cause a woman to feel ungainly and unattractive. She may say, "I can't even see my feet anymore" or "I feel as big as a house."

PSYCHOLOGIC TASKS OF THE MOTHER

Rubin (1984) identified the following developmental tasks of the mother:

1. *Ensuring safe passage through pregnancy, labor, and birth.* To meet this task she seeks competent prenatal care, practices good health behaviors and self-care activities, reads about childbirth, and gathers information.
2. *Seeking acceptance of this child by others.* The expectant woman seeks to gain support for the coming child from her partner and family. She will also work to help her other children accept the coming baby.
3. *Seeking of commitment and acceptance of self as mother to the infant (binding-in).* After she perceives fetal movement (quickening), the mother begins to form bonds of attachment to the child, and the child becomes more real. The woman may talk about the child as a separate person: "The baby was so active today! I don't think he (or she) appreciated the pizza last night."
4. *Learning to give of one's self on behalf of one's child.* The woman begins to develop patterns of self-denial and delayed personal gratification to meet the needs of her child. She may, for example, give up smoking or alcohol and make plans to adjust her personal schedule to spend more time with her child.

CRITICAL TERMS
FOR ANTEPARTAL ASSESSMENT

Gravida: Any pregnancy, regardless of duration.

Primigravida: A woman who is pregnant for the first time.

Multigravida: A woman who is pregnant with her second child or any subsequent pregnancy.

Para: Birth after 20 weeks' gestation, regardless of whether the infant is alive or dead.

Multipara: A woman who has had two or more births at more than 20 weeks' gestation.

Note: In clinical practice caregivers often refer to a woman who is pregnant for the first time as a *primip* (short for primipara). The correct term would actually be *nullipara*, but it is seldom used. A woman becomes a primipara after she has had one birth of more than 20 weeks' gestation. Thus the term could be used on postpartum.

Preterm labor: Labor that occurs after 20 weeks but before the completion of 37 weeks of gestation.

Stillbirth: A fetus born dead after 20 weeks' gestation.

PRENATAL CLIENT HISTORY
Gravida/Para Notation

- Systems are used to describe a woman's pregnancy history.
- Example: Woman pregnant for the first time is gravida 1, para 0 (or G1 P0).
- Example: Woman pregnant for the second time who has one living child born at term and had one miscarriage (also called spontaneous abortion) is gravida 2 para 1 abortion 1 (G2 P1 Ab1).
- Some agencies use a more detailed approach using term, preterm, abortions, and living children.
- Gravida means the same as in the previous example; instead of para as it is traditionally defined, the focus is on the number of infants born and is further divided to identify the number of term, preterm, abortions, and living children.

- Example: Woman pregnant for the first time is gravida 1 para 0000 (sometimes listed as 10000, 1 for gravida, 0000 for para).
- Example: Second woman (described earlier) would be gravida 2 para 1011, for one term infant, no preterm, one abortion, one living child (21011).

Current Pregnancy

- *LMP*—that is, first day of last normal menstrual period (helps to date pregnancy)
- Presence of any problems or complications such as bleeding
- Any discomforts, concerns, or questions

History of Past Pregnancies

- Information includes number of pregnancies, abortions (spontaneous or therapeutic), living children, and complications. (This history helps caregivers avoid unintentionally hurtful comments and alerts them to potential problems. For example, a woman with a history of preterm labor is at increased risk for preterm labor.)

Gynecologic History

- Obtain detailed gynecologic history.
- Include information on contraceptive history (e.g., an intrauterine device in place is usually removed because it could cause spontaneous abortion).
- Include history of sexually transmitted infections.
- Include history of abnormal Pap smears.

Current and Past Medical History

- This history provides information about woman's general state of health and health habits, as well as any medical-surgical conditions that might affect the pregnancy, such as diabetes, heart disease, and sickle cell anemia.
- Note use of alcohol, cigarettes, or drugs; exposure to teratogens; allergies; current medications; blood type and Rh factor; and record of immunizations, especially rubella.

Religious/Cultural/Occupational History

Information is obtained about any religious preferences, cultural influences, and any workplace hazards.

High-Risk Pregnancy

Certain factors in the woman's history place her at increased risk for complications during her current pregnancy. These factors include smoking, maternal age less than 20, previous preterm birth, and so forth. Preexisting medical conditions such as maternal diabetes automatically place the woman in a higher risk category. After the history is obtained, most agencies use a form to rate the number of risk factors and obtain a score. *Women who fall into a high-risk category are monitored more closely for potential complications.*

Partner's History

Information is obtained about the partner's age; health; current and past medical history; use of substances including alcohol, cigarettes, social drugs, and so forth; blood type and Rh factor; occupation; and attitude about the pregnancy.

INITIAL PRENATAL PHYSICAL EXAMINATION

The nurse is responsible for the following assessments at the initial prenatal examination:

- Vital signs, including temperature, pulse, respirations, and BP (some agencies omit temperature).
- Height and weight.
- Urinalysis (to detect proteinuria, glycosuria, hematuria, and so forth).
- Blood for complete blood count, including Hct (to detect anemia) and differential, Venereal Disease Research Laboratories, ABO and Rh typing, Rubella titer (to detect whether the woman is immune to German measles), sickle cell screen for clients of African descent, and other lab tests as ordered. Human immunodeficiency virus screen and drug screen are offered to all women, as is prenatal screening for cystic fibrosis.

- First-trimester ultrasound assessment of the thickness of the fetal nuchal fold (nuchal translucency) offered in combination with a serum screen of pregnancy-associated plasma protein A offered at initial visit. Used to help detect Down syndrome, trisomy 18, some heart defects, and other abnormalities.

The nurse then remains in the room to assist the examiner with the physical exam, including the pelvic exam.

Critical Elements of Initial Prenatal Examination

1. **Skin.** Color noted (to detect anemia, cyanosis, and jaundice); edema noted (may be normal or could indicate preeclampsia); changes normally associated with pregnancy noted, such as chloasma (melasma), linea nigra, and spider nevi.
2. **Neck.** Thyroid assessed (may enlarge slightly during pregnancy); marked enlargement, nodules, and so forth could indicate hyperthyroidism or goiter and are assessed further.
3. **Lungs.** Inspection, palpation, and auscultation should be normal, with no adventitious sounds.
4. **Breasts.** Inspection and palpation performed. Normal changes of pregnancy noted. Orange-peel skin and palpable nodule suggest possible carcinoma; redness indicates mastitis.
5. **Heart.** Rate, rhythm, and heart sounds noted; should be normal. Short systolic murmur common because of increased blood volume.
6. **Abdomen.** Inspection and palpation performed. Liver and spleen not palpable. Shows changes of pregnancy including enlargement and striae.
   a. *Fundus* (upper portion of uterus) palpable as follows:
      - 10–12 weeks: slightly above symphysis
      - 16 weeks: halfway between symphysis and umbilicus

- 20 weeks: at umbilicus
- 28 weeks: three finger breadths above umbilicus
- 36 weeks: just below ensiform cartilage

b. Fetal heartbeat auscultated as follows:
- 10–12 weeks: heard with Doppler (rate 110–160 beats per minute)
- 17–20 weeks: heard with stethoscope

c. Examiner can palpate fetal movement at 20 weeks' gestation.

7. **Reflexes.** At least brachial and patellar assessed. Hyperreflexia could indicate developing preeclampsia. (See Procedures: Assessing Deep Tendon Reflexes and Clonus. Preeclampsia is discussed in Chapter 2.)

8. **Pelvic exam.** External and internal genitals inspected, Pap obtained; gonorrhea culture (and sometimes chlamydia screen) obtained; changes of pregnancy noted, including Chadwick's sign and Goodell's sign. Uterine size evaluated to determine whether size seems appropriate for length of gestation. Ovaries palpated.

9. **Pelvic dimensions.** The following dimensions are considered necessary for vaginal birth (see Figures 1–1, 1–2, and 1–3).
- Pelvic inlet: Diagonal conjugate (extends from lower border of symphysis pubis to sacral promontory) at least 11.5 cm (Figure 1–1).
- Pelvic outlet: Anteroposterior diameter (from lower border of symphysis pubis to tip of sacrum) 9.5–11.5 cm (Figure 1–1).
- Pelvic outlet: Transverse diameter (measured by placing a fist between the ischial tuberosities) 8–10 cm (Figure 1–2).
- Subpubic angle: Obtained by palpating bony structure externally, normally 85–90 degrees (Figure 1–3).

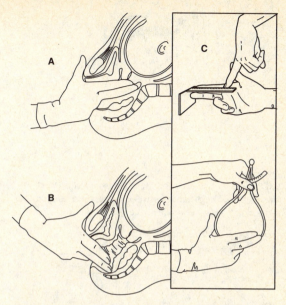

Figure 1–1 ■ Manual measurement of inlet and outlet.
A, Estimation of diagonal conjugate, which extends from the lower border of the symphysis pubis to the sacral promontory. **B,** Estimation of anteroposterior diameter of the outlet, which extends from the lower border of the symphysis pubis to the tip of the sacrum. **C,** Methods that may be used to check manual estimation of anteroposterior measurements.

- Mobility of coccyx assessed by pressing on coccyx; it should be mobile.
10. **Rectal exam.** Rashes, lumps, and hemorrhoids noted; woman with hemorrhoids should be assessed for problems with constipation.

DETERMINATION OF DUE DATE

The *due date* (date around which childbirth will occur), also called the estimated date of birth or estimated date

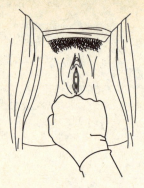

Figure 1–2 ■ Use of closed fist to measure outlet. Most examiners know the distance between the first and last proximal knuckles. If not, a measuring device can be used.

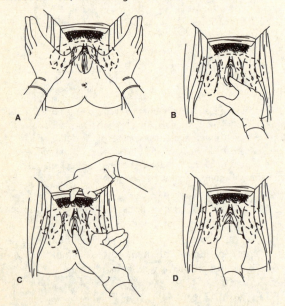

Figure 1–3 ■ Evaluation of outlet. A, Estimation of suprapubic angle. B, Estimation of length of pubic ramus. C, Estimation of depth and inclination of pubis. D, Estimation of contour of suprapubic angle.

of confinement, helps the caregiver determine if the fetus is growing appropriately. It also helps determine whether the start of labor occurs at the correct time or prematurely.

1. **Nägele's rule.** Due date is calculated using a formula called Nägele's rule. To use this formula, one begins with the first day of the woman's LMP, subtracts 3 months, and adds 7 days. For example

First day of LMP	November 21
Subtract 3 months	− 3 months
	August 21
Add 7 days	+ 7 days
Estimated date of birth	August 28

Note: Due date can also be calculated using a *gestational wheel.*

2. **Uterine assessment, or sizing the uterus.** A skilled examiner can determine by bimanual examination if the size of the uterus is appropriate for the weeks of pregnancy. This is an especially valuable technique in the first trimester.

3. **Measurement of fundal height.** After the first trimester the uterus is palpable in the abdomen. Its height—the distance from the top of the symphysis pubis to the top of the fundus—can be measured with a centimeter tape measure. Fundal height corresponds well with weeks of gestation, especially between 20 and 31 weeks. For example, 24 cm would suggest 24 weeks' gestation.

4. **Quickening (perception of fetal movement by the mother).** Quickening almost always occurs by 19–20 weeks' gestation. Because it may occur any time from 16–22 weeks, this is a less specific measure.

5. **Fetal heartbeat.** The heartbeat can be detected with a Doppler by 10–12 weeks' gestation and with a fetoscope by 19–20 weeks' gestation.

6. **Ultrasound.** This procedure can be used to detect a gestational sac in early pregnancy and to determine specific fetal measurements, such as biparietal diameter, which are useful in determining gestational age.

FREQUENCY OF PRENATAL VISITS IN NORMAL PREGNANCY

- Every 4 weeks for first 28 weeks of gestation
- Every 2 weeks to week 36
- After week 36, weekly until birth

INITIAL PSYCHOSOCIAL ASSESSMENT

The psychosocial assessment helps to determine the woman's attitude about the pregnancy, teaching needs, support systems available to her, cultural or religious preferences, economic status, and living conditions. The following critical nursing assessments require further evaluation and intervention:

- Marked anxiety, apathy, fear, or anger about the pregnancy
- Isolated home environment without support systems available
- Language barriers
- Cultural practices that might endanger the child
- Long-term family problems
- Unstable or limited economic status; limited prenatal care
- Crowded or questionable living conditions

CARE DURING REGULAR PRENATAL VISITS

Critical Nursing Responsibilities

1. **Weigh woman.** During the first trimester a woman gains 3.5–5 lb; during the second and third trimesters she gains about 1 lb per week. Thus, when she is seen every 4 weeks, a 4-lb gain is normal. *Be alert for:*
   - Inadequate gain: Evaluate reasons; counsel on nutrition.

- Excessive gain: Often first sign of developing preeclampsia, a major complication of pregnancy (see Chapter 2 for further assessments).

2. **Monitor vital signs.** Pulse may increase slightly. BP usually decreases slightly toward midpregnancy and gradually returns to normal. Temperature and respirations may be omitted unless adverse symptoms are present. *Be alert for*:
   - Rapid pulse: Could indicate anxiety or cardiac problem. Report findings.
   - Elevated BP: A cardinal sign of preeclampsia (see Chapter 2 for further assessments).

3. **Assess for edema.** Some edema of ankles and feet is normal, especially in the last trimester. *Be alert for*:
   - Edema of hands, face, and legs—usually related to weight gain and may indicate preeclampsia (see Chapter 2 for further assessments).

4. **Collect dipstick urine specimen.** *Be alert for*:
   - Proteinuria 1+: Could indicate preeclampsia (see Chapter 2).
   - Glycosuria: Slight glycosuria may be normal but requires further assessment. It might indicate gestational diabetes mellitus (see Chapter 2 for further assessments).

5. **Glucose screen.** Between 24 and 28 weeks' gestation, a 50-g, 1-hour oral glucose screen is done. Plasma glucose levels of 130–140 mg/dL indicate the need to complete a 3-hour oral glucose tolerance test. Women with risk factors (age over 40; family history of diabetes; a prior macrosomic, malformed, or stillborn infant; obesity; hypertension; or glycosuria) should be screened as soon as feasible early in pregnancy (American Diabetes Association).

6. **Danger signs of pregnancy.** Ask whether the woman is experiencing any of the danger signs of pregnancy (see following discussion).

7. **Discomforts.** Ask about the common discomforts of pregnancy and provide appropriate information (see pages 21–24).

A certified nurse-midwife, nurse practitioner, or physician completes remainder of exam, which includes the following:

1. Review of history and findings.
2. Assessment of uterine size, measurement of fundal height.
3. Assessment of fetal heartbeat (normal 110–160 beats per minute) and position.
4. Assessment of deep tendon reflexes and clonus (see Procedures: Assessing Deep Tendon Reflexes and Clonus, pp. 315–318).
5. Vaginal exam not repeated until last weeks of pregnancy.

DANGER SIGNS OF PREGNANCY AND POSSIBLE CAUSES

Table 1–1 identifies the danger signs of pregnancy and the possible causes. These findings indicate a potentially serious problem and require further assessment. The nurse reviews these signs and stresses to the woman the importance of reporting them immediately if they occur. *Discuss them at each prenatal visit.*

PRENATAL NUTRITION

1. Recommended dietary allowance for most nutrients increases.
2. For a woman of normal prepregnant weight, the recommended weight gain is 25–35 lb (11.4–15.9 kg).
3. Pattern of weight gain
   - First trimester: 3.5–5 lb (1.6–2.3 kg).
   - Second and third trimesters: About 1 lb per week.
   - Caloric increase: Only 300 kcal day. Idea that woman is "eating for two" can lead to excessive weight gain.
4. Overweight women should not diet during pregnancy.

Table 1–1   Danger Signs in Pregnancy

The woman should report the following danger signs in pregnancy immediately:

Danger Sign	Possible Cause
1. Sudden gush of fluid from vagina	Premature rupture of membranes
2. Vaginal bleeding	Abruptio placentae, placenta previa, lesions of cervix or vagina, "bloody show"
3. Abdominal pain	Premature labor, abruptio placentae
4. Temperature above 38.3°C (101°F) and chills	Infection
5. Dizziness, blurring of vision, double vision, spots before eyes	Hypertension, preeclampsia
6. Persistent vomiting	Hyperemesis gravidarum
7. Severe headache	Hypertension, preeclampsia
8. Edema of hands, face, legs, and feet	Preeclampsia
9. Muscular irritability, convulsions	Preeclampsia, eclampsia
10. Epigastric pain	Preeclampsia-ischemia in major abdominal vessels
11. Oliguria	Renal impairment, decreased fluid intake
12. Dysuria	Urinary tract infection
13. Absence of fetal movement	Maternal medication, obesity, fetal death

5. In second and third trimesters, further evaluation is indicated for the following:
   - Inadequate gain (less than 2.2 lb [1 kg]/month).
   - Excessive gain (more than 6.6 lb [3 kg]/month).

Critical Information in Counseling about Nutrition

1. Stress the use of the Food Guide Pyramid, including the following:

   Bread, cereal, rice, and pasta: Adults need 6–11 servings (1 serving = 1 slice bread, 1 oz dry cereal, ½ hamburger roll, 1 tortilla, ½ cup pasta, ½ cup rice or grits).

Vegetable group: Adults need 3–5 servings (1 serving = ½ cup cooked vegetables; 1 cup raw vegetables).

Fruit group: Adults need 2–4 servings (1 serving = 1 medium-sized piece of fruit, ½ cup of juice). One of those servings should be a good source of vitamin C.

Milk, yogurt, cheese group: Adults need 2–3 servings (1 serving = 1 cup milk or yogurt, 1.5 oz hard cheese, 2 cups cottage cheese, 1 cup pudding made with milk).

Meat, poultry, fish, dry beans, eggs, and nuts group: Adults need 2–3 servings (1 serving = 2 oz cooked lean meat, poultry, or fish; 2 eggs; ½ cup cooked legumes [kidney, lima, garbanzo, or soy beans, split peas, etc.]; 6 oz tofu; 2 oz nuts or seeds; 4 T peanut butter).

Fats, oils, sweets: Use sparingly.

2. To increase diet by 300 kcal, woman should add 2 milk servings and 1 meat or meat alternative.

3. To get maximum benefit without additional calories, use low-fat dairy products, lean cuts of meat, low-fat cooking methods such as baking or broiling instead of frying, and so forth.

4. Limit extras that have little nutritional value and are high in sugar or fat, such as doughnuts, chips, candy, mayonnaise, and so forth.

Nutrition for the Pregnant Adolescent

1. If adolescent is less than 4 years postmenarche, her nutritional needs include the increase for pregnancy (300 kcal) plus the intake necessary for her anticipated weight gain developmentally during the year she is pregnant.

2. Adolescent diets tend to be deficient in iron and calcium. Iron supplements are used and iron-rich foods are encouraged (see following discussion of nutrition for the woman with anemia). Calcium supplements may be necessary, usually 1,200 mg daily.

3. Folic acid supplements are given.

4. Many adolescents have a better diet than believed. Thus, their eating patterns over several days, not simply one day, should be assessed.

Nutrition for the Pregnant Vegetarian

Lacto-ovovegetarians include milk, dairy products, and eggs in their diet. Some also include fish and poultry. *Lactovegetarians* include dairy products but no eggs. *Vegans* are "pure" vegetarians who do not eat any food from animal sources.

If her diet permits, a woman can obtain adequate complete proteins from dairy products and eggs. Pure vegans must use complementing proteins such as unrefined grains (brown rice, whole wheat), legumes (beans, split peas, lentils), and nuts and seeds (in large quantities). Vegans should take a daily supplement of 4 g of vitamin B_{12}. Vegetarian diets also tend to be low in iron and zinc, and supplementation is often necessary.

Nutrition for the Woman with Anemia

To correct iron deficiency anemia, the woman will be given iron supplements. The nurse should explain to her that she can also help herself with the following dietary practices:

- Regularly eat meat, poultry, and fish, which are good sources of iron.
- Consume iron-fortified cereals and breads.
- Take vitamin C with meals to increase iron absorption. Good sources of vitamin C include citrus fruits, strawberries, tomatoes, cantaloupe, broccoli, peppers, and potatoes.
- Select iron-rich vegetables such as spinach, broccoli, dandelion greens, and other green leafy vegetables.
- Use iron pots and pans for cooking.

RELIEF OF THE COMMON DISCOMFORTS OF PREGNANCY

Nausea and Vomiting ("Morning Sickness")

- Avoid odors or factors that trigger nausea.
- Eat dry toast or crackers before rising.

- Have small but frequent dry meals with fluids between meals.
- Avoid greasy or highly seasoned foods.
- Drink carbonated beverages or herbal teas (e.g., peppermint, chamomile, spearmint).
- Women may benefit from acupressure wrist bands or acupressure to appropriate pressure points.

Urinary Frequency
- Increase daytime fluid intake; void when the urge is felt.
- Decrease fluid only in the evening to decrease nocturia.

Fatigue
- Plan time for a daily nap or rest period.
- Go to bed earlier.
- Seek family assistance with tasks so more time is available to rest.

Breast Tenderness
- Wear a well-fitting, supportive bra.

Increased Vaginal Discharge
- Bathe daily, but avoid douching, nylon underpants, and pantyhose.
- Wear cotton underpants.

Nasal Stuffiness and Epistaxis
- May be unresponsive; cool-air vaporizer may help.
- Avoid nasal sprays and decongestants.

Ptyalism
- Use astringent mouthwash, chew gum, or suck hard candy.

Pyrosis (Heartburn)
- Eat small, frequent meals; avoid overeating or lying down after eating.
- Use low-sodium antacids; avoid sodium bicarbonate.

Ankle Edema
- Dorsiflex foot frequently; elevate legs when sitting or resting.
- Avoid tight garters or constricting bands.

Varicose Veins
- Wear supportive hose and elevate feet frequently.
- Avoid crossing legs at knees, prolonged standing, and garters.

Constipation
- Increase fluid in diet. (Drink at least eight 8-oz glasses daily.)
- Increase fiber. (Increase fruits and vegetables to 6 servings; choose fresh fruit when possible, and include prunes or prune juice; increase grains to 6 servings and choose unrefined grains, such as whole wheat, brown rice, and bran; include legumes in place of meat.)
- Increase daily exercise to promote peristalsis.

Hemorrhoids
- Avoid constipation and straining to defecate.
- Reinsert into rectum if necessary; treat with topical anesthetics, warm soaks, sitz baths, or ice packs.

Backache
- Use good body mechanics; do pelvic tilt exercises regularly.
- Avoid uncomfortable working heights, high-heeled shoes, lifting heavy loads, and fatigue.

Leg Cramps
- Practice dorsiflexing foot to stretch affected muscle.
- Apply heat to affected muscle.

Faintness
- Avoid prolonged standing in warm area.
- Rise slowly from resting position.

Dyspnea

- Use proper posture when sitting or standing.
- Sleep propped up with pillows if problem occurs at night.

Difficulty Sleeping

- Drink a warm (caffeine-free) beverage before bed.
- Use pillows to provide support for back, between legs, or under upper arm when in a side-lying position.

Flatulence

- Chew food thoroughly and avoid gas-forming food.
- Exercise regularly and maintain normal bowel habits.

Carpal Tunnel Syndrome

- Avoid aggravating hand movements; use splint as prescribed.
- Elevate affected arm.

Monitoring Fetal Activity

- Vigorous fetal activity indicates fetal well-being, whereas a marked decrease in fetal activity may indicate fetal compromise and requires immediate evaluation. Fetal activity may be affected by drugs, cigarette smoking, sound, fetal sleep periods, blood glucose levels, and time of day. It has become accepted practice to teach pregnant women to monitor fetal activity daily beginning at about 27 weeks' gestation.
- The Cardiff Count-to-Ten is a frequently used method to evaluate fetal movement. To complete this self-assessment, the woman begins counting at a specified time daily and counts until 10 fetal movements have occurred. She should contact her caregiver if there are fewer than 10 movements in 3 hours or if it takes much longer each day to note 10 movements. The caregiver will probably order a nonstress test (NST).

BATHING

- Daily bathing, by shower or in a tub, is appropriate. The woman should take care to avoid slipping, especially because of her changed center of gravity. A rubber tub mat helps prevent falls.

- Tub baths are contraindicated in the presence of ruptured membranes or vaginal bleeding to avoid introducing infection.

EMPLOYMENT

Major problems with employment during pregnancy include exposure to fetotoxic hazards, excessive physical strain, overfatigue, medical or pregnancy-related complications, and, in later pregnancy, difficulty with occupations involving balance. Advise the woman who continues working to use breaks and lunch for rest, preferably on her side. Women who stand in place for long periods should dorsiflex their feet and walk around periodically to avoid problems with varicose veins, phlebitis, and edema.

TRAVEL

If no complications exist, there are no restrictions on travel. Travel by plane or train is preferable for long distances. The woman should walk about periodically to avoid phlebitis. If traveling by car she should plan to stop every 2 hours and walk around for 10 minutes. Seat belts should be worn with the lap belt positioned under the abdomen.

EXERCISE

- Exercise (at least 30 minutes of moderate exercise) is recommended daily or at least most days of the week. Swimming, cycling, walking, and cross-country skiing are good choices.
- Pregnancy is not the time to learn a new or strenuous sport.
- A pregnant woman should wear a supportive bra and appropriate shoes, should avoid hyperthermia, and should take fluids liberally to avoid dehydration.
- The woman should modify the intensity of her exercise based on her symptoms and should stop when she becomes fatigued.

- To avoid supine hypotensive syndrome, she should not lie flat on her back to exercise after the first trimester.
- Dizziness, extreme shortness of breath, tingling and numbness, palpitations, abdominal pain, vaginal bleeding, and abrupt cessation of fetal movement should be reported to her caregiver.

Exercises in Preparation for Childbirth

Teach abdominal tightening; partial, bent-knee sit-ups; Kegel exercises; and tailor sitting.

SEXUAL ACTIVITY

- Change in desire is normal and may vary according to trimester.
- In the first trimester, fatigue, nausea, and breast tenderness may lead to decreased desire in some women. The second trimester may be a time of increased desire, whereas the third trimester may also be a time of decreased desire.
- A woman should avoid lying flat on her back for intercourse after the fourth month to avoid vena caval (aortocaval) syndrome. If that position is preferred, she should place a pillow under her right hip to displace the uterus. Change in position, such as side-lying, female superior, or vaginal rear entry, may become necessary as her uterus enlarges.
- In the last weeks of pregnancy, orgasms may be more intense and may be followed by uterine cramping.
- *Stress that sexual intercourse is contraindicated once the membranes are ruptured or in the presence of vaginal bleeding to avoid introducing infection.* Women with a history of preterm labor may be advised to avoid intercourse in the third trimester because the oxytocin released with orgasm or with breast stimulation may trigger contractions. Couples who engage in anal intercourse should avoid going from anal penetration to vaginal penetration because of the risk of introducing infection.

- Men may notice a change in their level of desire, too. If a man feels the desire for further sexual release he may need to masturbate, either with his partner or in private.
- The couple can also be encouraged to explore other methods of expressing intimacy and affection, such as stroking, cuddling, and kissing.

MEDICATIONS, SMOKING, AND ALCOHOL

- Women should avoid taking medication—both prescribed and over-the-counter medication—when pregnant. If the need for medication arises, the woman should make certain her caregiver knows she is pregnant.
- Smoking is related to lower birth weight infants and to preterm labor. Women should avoid it as much as possible.
- Alcohol has been linked to neurologic deficits in newborns and to low birth weight. Heavy drinking may lead to fetal alcohol syndrome. Because it is not clear how much alcohol is problematic, alcohol should be avoided completely. Women should also avoid cocaine, crack, marijuana, and all social and street drugs during pregnancy.

CHARTING

Most prenatal records are composed of a series of columns for making notations succinctly. These columns include height, weight, BP, urine, fetal heart rate (FHR), fundal height, edema, fetal movement, clonus, and so forth. Notations should be made in the comments section about any deviations from normal, about any teaching done, and about any special procedures. Charting on the prenatal record tends to be especially succinct, as the following example demonstrates:

> Basic four food groups and caloric increases for pregnancy discussed. Handout on prenatal nutrition reviewed and given to client. Reports she is taking prenatal vitamins regularly. States that nausea has decreased and she

is walking 2 miles/four times/week. No problems or distress. Will call if symptoms develop. A. Montoya, RN

ASSESSMENT OF FETAL WELL-BEING
Ultrasound
- Obstetric ultrasound is done either transvaginally or transabdominally, depending on the timing in pregnancy and the purpose of the ultrasound. Ultrasound is generally painless and nonradiating to the woman and fetus; it has no known harmful effects. Serial studies can be done for assessment and comparison.
- Ultrasound can be used for early identification of pregnancy (as early as the fifth or sixth week after LMP); for identification of more than one fetus; to measure biparietal diameter; to detect fetal anomalies, *hydramnios* (excess amniotic fluid), or *oligohydramnios* (too little fluid); to locate and grade the placenta; and to observe FHR, movement, respirations, position and presentation, or fetal death.

Nonstress Test
1. The NST is used to assess fetal status using an electronic fetal monitor to observe baseline variability and acceleration of FHR with movement. FHR accelerations indicate that the fetal central and autonomic nervous systems have not been affected by decreased oxygen to the fetus.
2. **Procedure.** The NST may be done in a clinic or an inpatient setting. Women are requested to be nonfasting and to have refrained from recent cigarette smoking because this can adversely affect test results. The woman is placed in semi-Fowler's position, in a side-lying position, or in a reclining chair. Two belts are placed on the woman's abdomen: One records the FHR; the other records uterine or fetal movement. The fetal monitor begins recording activity. The woman is instructed to press a button on the monitor (or on the uterine belt) each time she feels the fetus move. This causes a mark on the

tracing paper. An assessment can then be made as to whether FHR accelerations occurred with each fetal movement.

3. Interpretation of NST results
   - **Reactive test** shows two or more accelerations of 15 beats per minute, lasting 15 seconds or more, over a period of 20 minutes (Figure 1–4).
   - **Nonreactive test** is one that lacks sufficient FHR accelerations over a 40-minute period (Figure 1–5).
   - **Unsatisfactory test** is one in which data cannot be interpreted or there is inadequate fetal activity.

4. A reactive NST usually indicates fetal well-being, and the test does not need to be repeated for a week. A nonreactive NST indicates the need for further testing.

5. **Nursing interventions.** The nurse explains the procedure, administers the NST, interprets the results, and reports the findings to the physician or certified nurse-midwife. If the fetus is not moving well, it is sometimes helpful to have the mother drink a glass of juice to increase her blood glucose level. This seems to result in increased fetal activity.

Note: If any decelerations in FHR occur during the procedure, the physician or nurse-midwife should be notified for further evaluation of fetal status.

Vibroacoustic Stimulation (VAS)

1. *Vibroacoustic stimulation* (VAS, also called fetal acoustic stimulation test or vibroacoustic stimulation test) is an application of sound and vibration to the mother's abdomen to stimulate movement in the fetus.

2. VAS is often used to improve the specificity and efficiency of interpretation of FHR monitoring patterns because a nonreactive NST may occur simply because the fetus is in a sleep cycle.

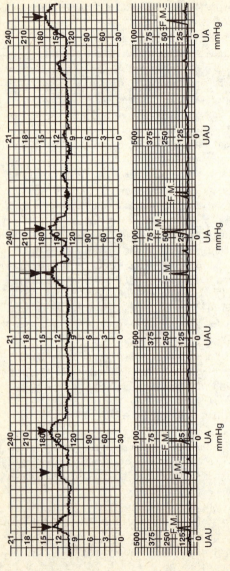

Figure 1–4 ■ Example of a reactive nonstress test. The top portion of the strip is a recording of the fetal heart rate. Note that most of the fetal heart rate tracing is relatively straight, with some areas that rise from this relatively straight line. These are accelerations. Each small square of the graph paper equals 10 seconds, so each of the indicated accelerations is more than 15 seconds in length. Each of the identified accelerations occurs with a fetal movement (F.M.), which is recorded on the bottom portion of the strip. The criteria for a reactive nonstress test have been met on this tracing. UA, umbilical artery.

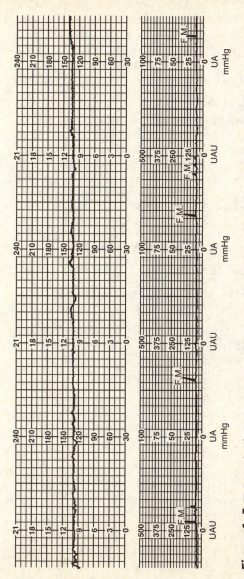

Figure 1–5 ▓ Example of a nonreactive nonstress test. There are no accelerations of the fetal heart rate with the episodes of fetal movement indicated on the bottom portion of the strip. F.M., fetal movement; UA, umbilical artery.

3. A device is used to deliver 1–3 seconds of sound to the fetus to change the fetal behavioral state, thereby accelerating the FHR.
4. The typical VAS response of a healthy term fetus shows at least a 10 beats per minute rise in baseline, occurring within 10 seconds and lasting 5–10 minutes.

Biophysical Profile

The biophysical profile is a collection of information about selected fetal measurements and assessments of the fetus and the amniotic fluid. It includes five variables: fetal breathing movements, body movement, tone, FHR activity, and amniotic fluid volume. Table 1–2 identifies scoring techniques and interpretation. Table 1–3 outlines a management protocol.

Table 1–2   Criteria for Normal and Abnormal Assessments

Component	Normal (Score = 2)	Abnormal (Score = 0)
Fetal breathing movements	Greater than or equal to 1 episode of rhythmic breathing lasting 30 seconds within 30 minutes	Less than or equal to 30 sec of breathing in 30 minutes
Gross body movements	Greater than or equal to 3 discrete body or limb movements in 30 minutes (episodes of active continuous movement considered as single movement)	Less than or equal to 2 movements in 30 minutes
Fetal tone	Greater than or equal to 1 episode of extension of a fetal extremity with return to flexion, or opening or closing of hand	No movements or extension/flexion
Reactive nonstress test	Greater than or equal to 2 accelerations of greater than or equal to 15 beats per min for 15 seconds in 20–40 minutes	0 or 1 acceleration in 20–40 minutes
Amniotic fluid volume	Single vertical pocket greater than 2 cm or sum of 4 pockets greater than 5 cm	Largest single vertical pocket less than or equal to 2 cm. Total volume less than 5 cm

Table 1–3 BPP Interpretation and Recommended Management

Test Score	Interpretation	Perinatal Mortality within 1 Week without Intervention	Management
10/10	Normal non-asphyxiated fetus	Less than 1/1000	No fetal indication for intervention; repeat test weekly except in diabetic client and pregnancies that are post-term (twice weekly)
8/10 (normal fluid); 8/8 if no NST done	Risk of fetal asphyxia extremely rare	Less than 1/1000	Same as above
8/10 (abnormal fluid)	Chronic fetal asphyxia suspected	89/1000	Ensure birth
6/10	Possible fetal asphyxia	89/1000	If amniotic fluid volume abnormal, birth indicated
			If normal fluid at 36 weeks with favorable cervix, ensure birth
			If repeat test less than or equal to 6, ensure birth
			If repeat test greater than 6, observe and repeat per protocol
4/10	Probable fetal asphyxia	91/1000	Repeat testing same day; if BPP score less than or equal to 6, ensure birth
2/10	Almost certain fetal asphyxia	125/1000	Ensure birth
0/10	Certain fetal asphyxia	600/1000	Ensure birth

BPP, biophysical profile; NST, nonstress test.

Amniotic Fluid Analysis (Amniocentesis)

- Amniotic fluid can be withdrawn through a needle inserted through the abdominal wall into the uterus and analyzed to obtain valuable information about fetal status. Amniotic fluid analysis provides genetic information about the fetus and can also be used to determine fetal lung maturity. (See Procedures: Assisting During Amniocentesis, pp. 321–323.)

- Fetal lung maturity can be ascertained by determining the ratio of the phospholipids lecithin and sphingomyelin, the *L/S ratio*. These are two components of *surfactant*, the substance that lowers the surface tension of the alveoli of the lungs when the newborn exhales, thereby preventing lung collapse. Early in pregnancy the sphingomyelin component is greater than the lecithin, so the lecithin-to-sphingomyelin (L/S) ratio is low. As pregnancy progresses, the lecithin increases. Fetal maturity is indicated by an L/S ratio of 2:1 or greater.

- Delayed lung maturation is often seen in infants born to diabetic mothers. Thus an L/S ratio of 3:1 or higher may be necessary in these infants to ensure lung maturity.

- *Phosphatidylglycerol*, another phospholipid, appears in the amniotic fluid after about 35 weeks' gestation, and the amount continues to increase to term.

REFERENCES

Rubin, R. (1984). *Maternal identity and the maternal experience.* New York: Springer.

2 THE AT-RISK ANTEPARTAL CLIENT

DIABETES MELLITUS

- Condition in which the pancreas does not produce enough insulin to allow necessary carbohydrate metabolism. Glucose does not enter the cells, and they become energy depleted.
- The physiologic changes of pregnancy can drastically alter insulin requirements.
  1. In the first half of pregnancy, maternal hormones stimulate increased insulin production by the pancreas and increased tissue response to insulin.
  2. In the second half of pregnancy, maternal hormones cause increased resistance to insulin. Concurrently, increased amounts of maternal glucose are being diverted to the fetus.
  3. Any diabetic potential may be influenced by this increased stress on the β-cells of the pancreas.
- Classification
  1. Formerly classified according to pharmacologic treatment as type I (insulin-dependent diabetes mellitus [IDDM]) and type II (non-insulin-dependent diabetes mellitus [NIDDM])
  2. Newer classification (based on cause) into four main categories: type 1, type 2, other specific types, and gestational diabetes mellitus (GDM)

Gestational Diabetes Mellitus

- GDM refers to diabetes that develops during pregnancy.

- All pregnant women, regardless of risk factors, should be screened for GDM.
  1. Testing is done at 24–28 weeks' gestation.
  2. 1-hour, 50-g oral glucose tolerance test (GTT) used.
  3. If plasma glucose is greater than or equal to 130–140 mg/dL, 3-hour oral glucose tolerance test indicated.
- GDM is diagnosed if two or more of the following values are equaled or exceeded:
  - Fasting: 95 mg/dL
  - 1 hour: 180 mg/dL
  - 2 hour: 155 mg/dL
  - 3 hour: 140 mg/dL
- Often, gestational diabetes can be managed with diet, although some women receive regular insulin as well.

Pregestational Diabetes Mellitus

- Diabetes mellitus (DM) present before conception.
- Changes in glucose metabolism that result with pregnancy can affect diabetic control and can contribute to possible accelerations of the vascular disease associated with DM.
- Infants of diabetic mothers (IDM) are at greater risk for mortality or morbidity than are infants of mothers without diabetes.
- Long-term (previous 4–8 weeks) glucose control is assessed by measuring glycohemoglobin (HbA_{1C}). Women with values greater than 10% are at increased risk of having an infant with a malformation.
- Maternal risks: *Hydramnios* (excessive volume of amniotic fluid), preeclampsia, ketoacidosis, fetal macrosomia (large-size infant) leading to *dystocia* (difficult labor), anemia, monilial vaginitis, urinary tract infection (UTI), and retinopathy.
- Fetal-neonatal risks: Intrauterine growth restriction (IUGR), macrosomia, hypoglycemia, respiratory distress syndrome, hyperbilirubinemia, and congenital anomalies.

Management of Diabetes Mellitus in Pregnancy

- Dietary regulation
  1. Caloric needs of pregnant women are not altered by diabetes—about 30 kcal/kg ideal body weight (IBW) during first trimester and 35 kcal/kg ideal body weight during second and third trimesters.
  2. Approximately 40%–46% of calories should come from complex carbohydrates, 12%–20% from protein, and 35%–40% from fat (Reece & Homko, 2008).
  3. These calories are divided among three meals and three snacks.
  4. Bedtime snack, which should contain both protein and complex carbohydrates, is most important because of the risk of hypoglycemia during the night.

- Glucose monitoring
  1. Weekly in-office assessment of fasting glucose levels and occasional postprandial checks are generally indicated.
  2. Home monitoring of blood glucose levels four to six times daily.
  3. Optimal range, fasting: below 95 mg/dL; 2 hours postprandial: less than 120 mg/dL (ADA, 2006).

- Insulin administration
  1. Insulin generally given in multiple injections using human insulin or a fast-acting human analog called Lispro.
  2. Four-dose approach often used with regular insulin or Lispro before each meal and NPH or Lente insulin added at bedtime (ACOG, 2005).
  3. Insulin may also be given by continuous subcutaneous infusion.
  4. Oral hypoglycemics are rarely used in pregnancy because they cross the placenta and have not been well studied. However, an oral agent, glyburide,

does not cross the placenta and is comparable to insulin without adverse effects on the mother or fetus. It is now sometimes used for women with GDM (ACOG, 2005; Perkins et al., 2007).

- Evaluation of fetal status
  1. Woman is taught to monitor daily fetal activity (see Chapter 1).
  2. Maternal serum alpha-fetoprotein (MSAFP) screening is done at 16–20 weeks' gestation because pregnancies complicated by diabetes are at increased risk of neural tube defects.
  3. Nonstress testing (NST) (see Chapter 1) is usually begun weekly at about 28 weeks. If evidence of IUGR, preeclampsia, oligohydramnios, or poorly controlled blood glucose exists, testing may begin as early as 26 weeks and may be done more often. Testing increases to twice weekly at 32 weeks. If a woman requires hospitalization, NSTs may be done daily.
  4. Ultrasound is done at 18 weeks to establish gestational age and diagnose multiple pregnancy or congenital anomalies. It is repeated at 28 weeks to monitor fetal growth for IUGR or macrosomia.
  5. Biophysical profiles are done in the third trimester to evaluate fetal well-being.

Antepartal Nursing Assessments for Diabetes Mellitus

- Assess urine for glucose and ketones at each prenatal visit.
- Assess results of blood glucose testing for women with diagnosed GDM or pregestational DM.
- Assess for any signs of UTI (dysuria, urgency, frequency, hematuria) or monilial vaginitis (excessive itching, curdy white discharge, dyspareunia).
- Assess woman's understanding of her condition, its treatment, and its implications.

- *Be alert for* hyperglycemia, hypoglycemia, evidence of infection, signs of vascular complications (ulceration of extremities, visual changes, and so forth).

Sample Nursing Diagnoses
- Health-seeking behaviors: information about GDM related to an expressed desire to learn more about the disease and its implications for the woman and her unborn child
- Interrupted family processes related to the need for hospitalization secondary to DM

Antepartal Nursing Interventions for Diabetes Mellitus
- Obtain serum glucose readings at the specified times (if woman is hospitalized).
- Administer insulin or Lispro as prescribed. Have a second nurse verify the dosage before administering the insulin.
- Monitor for signs of developing hypoglycemia (caused by too much insulin or too little food): sudden onset (minutes to ½ hour), sweating, periodic tingling, disorientation, shakiness, pallor, clammy skin, irritability, hunger, headache, and blurred vision.
  1. If untreated, convulsions and coma may develop.
  2. If they occur, immediately check woman's capillary glucose level (and teach her to do the same following discharge).
  3. Follow agency policy regarding procedure for correcting hypoglycemia for blood glucose less than 60 mg/dL. Administer 20 g carbohydrate, wait 20 minutes, and retest blood glucose. The necessary carbohydrate can be obtained by drinking 1 cup of skim milk, ½ cup orange or apple juice, or ½ cup regular soft drink or by eating four to six pieces of hard candy or 1 tablespoon of honey, corn syrup, or brown sugar (Cleveland Clinic, 2006). If the woman is not alert enough to swallow, give 1 mg glucagon subcutaneously or intramuscularly (IM) and notify physician.

- Monitor for signs of developing hyperglycemia (caused by too much food and too little insulin): typically slow onset, polyuria, polydipsia, dry mouth, increased appetite, fatigue, nausea, hot and flushed skin, rapid and deep breathing, abdominal cramps, acetone breath, headache, drowsiness, depressed reflexes, oliguria or anuria, and stupor or coma.
  1. If hyperglycemia is suspected, obtain frequent measures of blood glucose level; check urine for acetone.
  2. Administer prescribed amount of regular insulin subcutaneously, intravenously (IV), or by a combination of routes.
  3. Replace fluids; measure intake and output (I&O).
- Monitor fetal status including fetal heart rate (FHR) every 4 hours.
- Assist woman with determining fetal movement record daily.
- Do NSTs as ordered while woman is hospitalized.
- Provide appropriate American Diabetes Association (ADA) diet as indicated. Work with dietitian to ensure appropriate teaching is provided for the woman.
- Demonstrate procedure for home monitoring of blood glucose level:
  1. Wash hands thoroughly before finger puncture.
  2. Sides of fingers should be punctured (ends contain more pain-sensitive nerves).
  3. Hanging arm down for 30 seconds before puncture increases blood flow to fingers. Spring-loaded devices are available to make puncture easier.
  4. Cleanse finger with alcohol pad first and allow alcohol to air dry.
  5. Touch blood droplet, not finger, to test pad on strip. Droplet should completely cover the test pad.
  6. If using visual method, wait prescribed time and compare color to color chart. If using a glucose meter, follow directions for use exactly.

7. Record results and bring record sheet to each prenatal visit.
- Complete client teaching, including the following:
  1. Procedures for home glucose monitoring and insulin administration (if woman is not already familiar with them)
  2. Signs of hypoglycemia and required treatment
  3. Signs of hyperglycemia and required treatment
  4. American Diabetes Association diet
- Review the following critical aspects of the care you have provided:
  1. Have I administered the correct doses of insulin at the specified times after first determining blood glucose levels?
  2. Have I been alert for any signs of hypoglycemia or hyperglycemia?
  3. Have I monitored FHR and fetal activity carefully and discussed with the woman her perceptions of fetal activity?
  4. Have I assessed the woman's understanding of her DM and answered her questions? Have I given her opportunities to practice specific skills as necessary?
  5. Have I ensured that the woman is eating the appropriate meals?

Evaluation

- The woman is able to discuss her condition and its possible impact on her pregnancy.
- The woman participates in developing a healthcare regimen to meet her needs and follows it throughout pregnancy.
- The woman avoids developing hypoglycemia or hyperglycemia; if either of these does develop, therapy is successful in correcting it without complications.
- The woman gives birth to a healthy newborn.

PREECLAMPSIA-ECLAMPSIA DURING THE ANTEPARTAL PERIOD

- Preeclampsia-eclampsia is the most common hypertensive disorder in pregnancy.
- It is characterized by the development of hypertension and proteinuria after 20 weeks' gestation.

  (Note: Previously, edema was included as part of the definition, but it has been excluded because edema is such a common finding in normal pregnancy; however, sudden edema warrants evaluation.)

- The definition of preeclampsia is:
  1. A blood pressure (BP) of 140/90 mm Hg during the second half of pregnancy in a previously normotensive woman.
  2. These BP changes must be noted on at least two occasions greater than or equal to 6 hours apart for the diagnosis to be made.

- *Mild preeclampsia* is characterized by:
  1. BP of 140/90 or higher on two occasions at least 6 hours apart.
  2. Proteinuria of 1+ to 2+ on dipstick (between 300 mg/L and 1 g/L or less than 5 g in 24 hours).
  3. Although no longer considered diagnostic, generalized edema of the face, hands, legs, and ankles may occur. This is usually associated with a weight gain of more than 1 lb/week.

- *Severe preeclampsia* is characterized by:
  1. BP of 180/110 on two occasions at least 6 hours apart while the woman is on bed rest
  2. Proteinuria equal to or greater than 5 g in 24 hours (3+ to 4+ dipstick)
  3. Oliguria (urine output less than or equal to 500 mL/24 hours)
  4. Headache
  5. Blurred vision, *scotomata* (spots before the eyes), and retinal edema on funduscopy (retinas appear wet and glistening)

6. Pulmonary edema
7. Hyperreflexia
8. Irritability
9. Epigastric or right upper quadrant pain
10. Impaired liver function (elevated hepatic enzymes [ALT or AST])

- *Eclampsia* is characterized by:
  1. Grand mal seizure or coma.
  2. The woman may have just 1 seizure or from 2–20 or more.
  3. Symptoms may increase in severity: BP of 180/110 or higher, 4+ proteinuria, oliguria, or anuria, and increased neurologic symptoms such as decreased sensorium or coma.

- Maternal risks with preeclampsia-eclampsia
  1. Retinal detachment
  2. Central nervous system changes including hyper-reflexia and seizure
  3. HELLP syndrome (**h**emolysis, **e**levated **l**iver enzymes, and **l**ow **p**latelet count)
     (Note: Women who experience HELLP, a multiple organ failure syndrome, and their offspring have high morbidity and mortality rates.)

- Fetal-neonatal risks
  1. Prematurity.
  2. IUGR.
  3. Oversedation at birth because of maternal medications.
  4. Neonatal morbidity and mortality in women with severe preeclampsia are primarily related to the newborn's gestational age at birth.

Antepartal Management of Preeclampsia-Eclampsia

The only known cure for preeclampsia is birth of the infant.

Mild Preeclampsia

- May be managed at home if the woman's condition is stable, if she has a basic understanding of her condition, is cooperative, and knows when to call her doctor. Hospitalization may be necessary if signs and symptoms worsen.
- Promotion of good placental and renal perfusion
    1. Frequent rest periods during the day in a side-lying position.
    2. Specific guidelines regarding rest periods may be given, including the amount of time in each rest period, number of rest periods daily, and activities during the day that are advisable or should be avoided.
    3. The more specific the guidelines, the more likely that the woman will clearly understand the information and restrictions.
- Dietary modifications
    1. Diet should be high in protein (80–100 g/day, or 1.5 g/kg/day).
    2. Sodium intake should be moderate, not exceeding 6 g/day.
- Evaluation of fetal status
    1. NSTs done weekly or biweekly.
    2. Additional tests include serial ultrasounds to evaluate fetal growth, amniocentesis and biophysical profile to determine fetal maturity, a contraction stress test if NST results indicate a need, and Doppler velocimetry to screen for fetal compromise.
- Evaluation of maternal well-being
    1. Woman is seen every 1–2 weeks.
    2. Taught to identify signs of a worsening condition.
    3. Does daily home monitoring of her BP, weight, urine protein, and fetal movement.

Severe Preeclampsia

- Hospitalization necessary

- Promotion of maternal well-being
  1. Complete bed rest in left lateral position, which decreases pressure on vena cava, thereby increasing venous perfusion. Improved renal blood flow helps decrease angiotensin II levels, promotes diuresis, and lowers BP.
  2. High-protein, moderate-sodium diet is continued.
  3. The woman is weighed daily (to detect edema) and evaluated for evidence of a change in condition through assessment of BP, TPR deep tendon reflexes (DTRs) and clonus, edema (generalized and pitting), presence of headache, visual disturbances, and epigastric pain.
- Evaluation of laboratory data
  1. Daily hematocrit (rising value may be associated with decreasing vascular volume).
  2. Daily liver enzyme testing, including AST, ALT, LDH, bilirubin (a rise in these tests correlates with a worsening condition).
  3. Daily uric acid and blood urea nitrogen (reflect renal status).
  4. Platelet counts every 2–3 days if over 100,000/mm^3, or daily if under 100,000/mm^3.

     (Note: Platelet count may be included in preeclamptic or disseminated intravascular coagulation [DIC] screen, which also determines prothrombin time, partial thromboplastin time, and fibrinogen and fibrin split products.)

     Platelet transfusions are indicated if the platelet count is below 20,000/mm^3.
- Medication therapy
  1. Magnesium sulfate is the treatment of choice for preventing convulsion (see Drug Guide: Magnesium Sulfate, pp. 294–297).
  2. Sedation with phenobarbital 30–60 mg po q6h may be indicated. (Some physicians prefer diazepam [Valium].)

3. An antihypertensive such as intravenous hydralazine (Apresoline), intravenous labetalol (Normodyne), or oral nifedipine may be used for sustained systolic BP of 160–180 mm Hg or for diastolic pressure of 105–110 mm Hg or above (Sabai, 2007).
4. Betamethasone or dexamethasone is often administered to the woman whose fetus has an immature lung profile. Corticosteroids may also be beneficial in stabilizing women with HELLP syndrome. Fluid and electrolytes are replaced as necessary based on the status of the woman.

Eclampsia

- Actions taken to control seizure may include bolus of magnesium sulfate, sedatives if necessary, and Dilantin for seizure prevention.
- The therapies discussed previously are continued.
- The airway is maintained.
- The woman is monitored for pulmonary edema, which may be treated with furosemide (Lasix).
- Digitalis may be given for circulatory failure.
- The woman may be transferred to an intensive care unit.

Antepartal Nursing Assessments for Preeclampsia-Eclampsia

- Assess BP, pulse, and respirations q1–4h or more frequently if indicated.
- Assess temperature q4h unless elevated, then q2h.
- Assess FHR when maternal vital signs (VS) are assessed or continuously with an electronic fetal monitor.
- Assess intake and urinary output hourly or q4h. Output should be 700 mL/24 hours or greater, or at least 30 mL/hour.
- Assess urinary protein by dipstick of each urine specimen or a specimen from an indwelling bladder catheter.

- *Assessment technique:* A small sample of urine is collected in a urine specimen bottle or in a syringe. A few drops of urine are placed on the treated section of the dipstick. The color of the treated urine is compared with samples on the dipstick container after a specified period of time. See dipstick container for specific instructions.
- Assess urine specific gravity.
- Assess for evidence of edema.
- *Assessment technique:* Assess for pitting edema by pressing over bony areas, usually over the shin. After pressing with one fingertip for 3–5 seconds, evaluate the resulting depression. A slight depression is 1+; a pit 1 inch deep is 4+.
- Assess daily weight.
- *Assessment technique:* Use the same scales each day; weigh at the same time each day with the woman in similar clothing.
- Assess DTRs. Assess for clonus. (See Procedures: Assessing Deep Tendon Reflexes and Clonus, pp. 315–318.)
- Assess breath sounds; rales will be heard if pulmonary edema is developing.
- Assess laboratory results.
- Assess woman's coping responses, level of understanding regarding her condition, and emotional status.
- See Drug Guide: Magnesium Sulfate, pp. 294–297, for specific nursing assessments during magnesium sulfate therapy.
- *Be alert for* signs of worsening condition (increasing BP, headache, scotomata, increasing edema [especially of hands and face], disorientation, epigastric pain, pitting edema) and signs of magnesium toxicity (respirations less than 12–14/minute, diminished or absent reflexes, urine output less than 100 mL in 4-hour period).

Sample Nursing Diagnoses
- Deficient fluid volume related to fluid shift from intravascular to extravascular space secondary to vasospasm and endothelial injury

- Risk of injury related to convulsion secondary to cerebral edema

Antepartal Nursing Interventions for Preeclampsia-Eclampsia

If the woman is managed at home, do the following:

- Teach the woman and her support person how to assess BP. Include positioning and specifics of the procedure. Assist them in developing a chart to record the findings. Instruct them about findings that should be reported to the physician.
- Provide teaching about the rest period regimen. Explain the purpose of the side-lying position.

If the woman is hospitalized, do the following:

- Monitor maternal BP, pulse and respirations, DTRs and clonus, and FHR q2–4h.
- Monitor oral temperature q4h unless elevated, then q2h.
- Weigh daily.
- Monitor I&O. Output should be at least 30 mL/hour. Specific gravity readings greater than 1.040 indicate oliguria.
- Monitor urine for proteinuria and specific gravity with each voiding, or monitor hourly if an indwelling catheter is in place.
- Monitor for signs of worsening condition including headache, visual disturbances, epigastric pain, and change in level of consciousness at least q4h.
- Encourage woman to maintain a side-lying position.
- Provide emotional support and teaching about condition and treatment plan.
- Administer magnesium sulfate and other medications as ordered. Monitor for evidence of effectiveness or toxicity.
- Provide a quiet, restful environment with limited visitors.

- Pad side rails and take seizure precautions.
- Review the following aspects of the care you have provided:
  1. What is the woman's response to the medications? Am I seeing any potential side effects?
  2. Is there a change in her ability to talk? Does she seem more irritable or confused?
  3. Is she complaining of headache or other symptoms that indicate a worsening condition?
  4. Is the baby moving as much as previously? Is FHR in normal range (110–160 beats per minute)?
  5. Positioning on which side produces the best results in FHR? Urine output? What can I do to help the woman maintain that position? A back rub? Pillows?
  6. Have I taken necessary safety precautions, including padded side rails, quiet environment, and calcium gluconate (magnesium sulfate antagonist) available?

Sample Nurse's Charting

1600: BP stable at 142/96, P 88, R 18, T 98.4F. FHR 138. Lungs clear to auscultation. DTRs, patellar and brachial, 2+ with no clonus. Pitting edema 1+ in legs, some swelling of fingers—rings snug. Slight periorbital edema evident. Urine S.G. 1.034; hourly output 40 mL/hr through indwelling Foley catheter. 2+ proteinuria. Magnesium sulfate maintenance dose running at 2 g/hr per infusion pump. No edema, redness, or c/o discomfort at infusion site. Continuous EFM with FHR baseline 140–146. Accelerations of 20 bpm for 20 sec noted with fetal movement. No decelerations noted. Client drowsy, responsive, oriented. States she has a slight headache but denies epigastric pain or visual changes. Resting quietly on her L side. Side rails padded and up. T. Varagoor, RN

Evaluation

- The woman is able to explain preeclampsia-eclampsia, its implications for her pregnancy, the treatment regimen, and possible complications.
- The woman does not have any eclamptic convulsions.
- The woman and her caregivers detect any evidence of increasing severity of the disease or possible complications early so that appropriate treatment measures can be instituted.
- The woman gives birth to a healthy newborn.

PRETERM LABOR

- Labor that occurs between 20 and 37 completed weeks of gestation is referred to as *preterm labor (PTL)*.
- It may result from maternal factors such as cardiovascular or renal disease, preeclampsia, diabetes, abdominal surgery during pregnancy, a blow to the abdomen, uterine anomalies, cervical incompetence, diethylstilbestrol exposure, history of cone biopsy, and maternal infection.
- Fetal factors include multiple pregnancy, hydramnios, and fetal infection; placental factors include placenta previa and abruptio placentae.
- The major maternal risks involve psychologic stress related to the woman's concern for her unborn child and physiologic side effects of the drugs used to stop labor.
- Fetal-neonatal risks are those related to the effects of prematurity. Of these factors, the most critical one is the lack of development of the respiratory system.

Management of Preterm Labor

- Confirmation of diagnosis
  1. A diagnosis of PTL is made if the gestation is between 20 and 37 completed weeks, if there are documented uterine contractions (four in 20 minutes or eight in 60 minutes), and ruptured membranes.

2. If the membranes are not ruptured, one of the following must be present: 80% cervical effacement, documented cervical changes, or 2 cm dilatation.
- Tests to screen high-risk women for PTL:
  1. **Fetal fibronectin (fFN).** Fetal fibronectin is a protein normally found in fetal membranes and decidua early in pregnancy, but not between 18 and 36 weeks' gestation. A negative test between 22 and 37 weeks indicates low risk of preterm birth within 14 days (Ness, et al., 2007). A positive test puts the woman at increased risk of preterm labor. It is also associated with recent sexual intercourse, vaginal examination, bacterial vaginosis, and vaginal bleeding, and is not very specific in predicting imminent birth (Tekesin et al., 2005).
  2. **Transvaginal ultrasound (TVS).** Length of the cervix can be measured using an ultrasound probe inserted into the vagina. A cervical length less than 25 mm prior to term is abnormal (Iams & Romero, 2007). Any medical conditions that may contribute to PTL should be treated.
- Maternal infections such as bacterial vaginosis, trichomoniasis, *Chlamydia trachomatis,* UTI, and asymptomatic bacteria are associated with PTL, so it is important to diagnose and treat infections (Newton, 2005).
- Mild symptoms of PTL may be treated with bed rest and hydration per infusion.
- If labor continues or if symptoms are severe, tocolysis (use of medication to stop labor) is begun.
- Tocolytics currently used to arrest PTL include magnesium sulfate, β-adrenergic agonists (also called β-mimetics), prostaglandin synthetase inhibitors (e.g., indomethacin [Indocin]), and calcium channel blockers (e.g., nifedipine).
  1. Magnesium sulfate is effective and has fewer side effects than the β-adrenergics. A loading dose of

4–8 g is administered IV over 20–60 minutes. A maintenance dose of 2–4 g/hr via infusion pump is then used until contractions cease (Carey & Gibbs, 2008).

2. Maternal serum level of 4.8–9.6 mg/dL is the effective range for tocolysis (see Drug Guide: Magnesium Sulfate, pp. 294–297).

3. The β-mimetics used include ritodrine (Yutopar), which has been approved by the U.S. Food and Drug Administration (FDA), and terbutaline (Brethine), which is not approved by the U.S. Food and Drug Administration for use in PTL but has become increasingly popular because it is effective and less expensive than ritodrine. Terbutaline is administered IV until uterine activity ceases.

4. Nifedipine, a calcium channel blocker, is sometimes co-administered with terbutaline or ritodrine for increased effectiveness; however, nifedipine and magnesium sulfate should not be co-administered because doing so may result in dangerously low maternal calcium levels.

- Betamethasone, an antenatal corticosteroid, may be given to the mother to help promote fetal lung maturation.

Nursing Assessments for Preterm Labor

- Assess carefully for evidence of complications or side effects from tocolysis, including tachycardia, palpitations, nervousness, nausea and vomiting, headache, and hypotension.
- *Be alert for* evidence of pulmonary edema, the most serious complication. Signs include shortness of breath, chest tightness, dyspnea, rales, and rhonchi.
- Assess for symptoms of magnesium toxicity in women receiving magnesium sulfate, including respirations less than 12 per minute, diminished or absent DTRs, and urine output less than 100 mL in 4-hour period.

Sample Nursing Diagnoses

- Ineffective Individual Coping related to need for constant attention to pregnancy
- Acute pain related to uterine contractions
- Fear related to the risks of early labor and birth

Nursing Interventions for Preterm Labor
Home Care

- Instruct women at risk about the signs and symptoms of PTL, which include the following:
    1. Uterine contractions occurring q10min or more frequently.
    2. Mild menstrual-like cramps felt low in the abdomen or abdominal cramping with or without diarrhea.
    3. Feelings of pelvic pressure that may feel like the baby pressing down. The pressure may be constant or intermittent.
    4. Constant or intermittent low backache.
    5. A sudden change in vaginal discharge (an increase in amount or a change to more clear and watery or a pinkish tinge).
- Teach the at-risk woman to evaluate contraction activity once or twice daily.
    1. Instruct her to lie on her side and place her fingertips on the fundus of the uterus.
    2. She checks for contractions (hardening of the fundus) for about 1 hour.
    3. Occasional contractions are probably normal Braxton Hicks contractions.
- If the woman experiences contractions every 10 minutes or any of the previously identified signs of labor, instruct her to do the following:
    1. Empty her bladder and lie down, preferably on her left side.
    2. Drink three to four 8-oz cups of fluid.

3. Palpate for uterine contractions, and if contractions occur 10 minutes apart or less for 1 hour, notify her healthcare provider.
4. Soak in a warm tub bath with the abdomen completely submerged for 30 minutes.
5. Rest for 30 minutes after symptoms have subsided and gradually resume activity.
6. Call her healthcare provider if symptoms persist, even if uterine contractions are not palpable.

Hospital Care

- Encourage bed rest in a side-lying position as much as possible.
- Monitor BP, pulse, and respirations as ordered, especially when on tocolytic therapy.
- Maintain continuous electronic monitoring of FHR and uterine contractions if ordered (see Chapter 3) and evaluate results.
- Monitor I&O.
- Administer betamethasone as ordered (see Drug Guide: Betamethasone, pp. 287–289).
- Explain procedures to the woman and her partner; answer questions and provide emotional support.
- Review the following critical aspects of the care you have provided:
  1. What is the woman's response to the tocolysis? Is she showing any side effects of the medication?
  2. Is she still having contractions? Have they increased or lessened? Is she showing other signs of labor?
  3. What is the fetus's response?
  4. What position is most effective? Are there nursing measures I can use to help her tolerate the side-lying position and the effects of tocolysis?
  5. How is she coping emotionally? Have I spent enough time helping her to cope with the stress of the situation?

Evaluation

- The woman is able to discuss the cause, identification, and treatment of PTL.
- The woman can describe self-care measures and can identify characteristics that should be reported to her caregiver.
- The woman and her baby have a safe labor and birth.

PLACENTA PREVIA IN THE ANTEPARTAL PERIOD

- In placenta previa the placenta is implanted in the lower uterine segment instead of the upper portion of the uterus. As the lower uterine segment contracts and dilates in the later weeks of pregnancy, the villi are torn from the uterine wall and bleeding results.
- If the placenta previa is complete, the placenta totally covers the internal cervical os.
- In partial placenta previa, a portion of the os is covered.
- Maternal risks are related to the possibility of hemorrhage and to psychologic stress resulting from concern about fetal well-being.
- Fetal-neonatal risks are related to the extent of the placenta previa. If a severe bleeding episode occurs, the fetus often suffers nonreassuring fetal status. Fetal demise is also a possibility if the condition is not diagnosed in a timely manner.

Antepartal Management of Placenta Previa

- **Diagnosis.** Diagnosis is made based on a history of painless, bright-red vaginal bleeding, especially in the third trimester. The initial bleeding episode may be light but is often followed by more severe bleeding. Diagnosis is confirmed with ultrasound to localize the placenta.
- **Expectant management.** If less than 37 weeks' gestation, expectant management is used to delay birth to allow the fetus to mature. This includes
  1. Bed rest.
  2. No rectal or vaginal exams.

3. Monitoring of bleeding.
4. Ongoing assessment of fetal status with external monitor.
5. Monitoring of VS.
6. Laboratory evaluation (hemoglobin, hematocrit, Rh factor, urinalysis).
7. Two units of cross-matched blood kept available for transfusion.

- If the previa is partial or if the placenta is simply low lying, vaginal birth may be attempted.
- **Emergency management.** If severe bleeding occurs or evidence of nonreassuring fetal status develops, a cesarean is performed.

Antepartal Nursing Assessments for Placenta Previa

- Assess woman regularly for evidence of vaginal bleeding. If bleeding is present, note the amount and character.
- Assess for signs of shock if bleeding is present (decreased BP, increased pulse, cool clammy skin, pallor, decreased hematocrit, urine output less than 30 mL/hour).
- Assess for uterine contractility and signs of labor. *Word of caution:* Vaginal exams may trigger a major bleeding episode and are contraindicated.
- Assess woman's understanding of her condition, its implications, and treatment options.
- Assess fetal status. During bleeding episode, continuous electronic fetal monitoring is used; when no bleeding is present, an electronic fetal monitoring strip is run, usually q4h (timing may vary according to agency policy).

Sample Nursing Diagnoses

- Altered tissue perfusion (placental) related to blood loss
- Fear related to concern for own personal well-being and that of the baby

Antepartal Nursing Interventions for Placenta Previa

- Carry out ongoing monitoring of maternal and fetal status including VS, evidence of bleeding, urinary output, electronic monitor tracing, and signs of labor.
- Explain procedures to woman and her family.
- Administer IV fluids or blood products as ordered.
- Review the following critical aspects of care you have provided:
  1. Have I questioned the woman about bleeding? If bleeding is present, have I assessed quantity carefully?
  2. Have I carefully monitored fetal status? Any signs of tachycardia? Decelerations?
  3. Have I been alert for any changes in the woman's status? Any signs of labor? Any changes she has noted?
  4. Have I implemented measures to help the woman be comfortable on bed rest—back rubs, positioning with pillows, diversionary activities?

Evaluation

- The woman's condition remains stable, or bleeding is detected promptly and therapy is begun.
- The woman and her baby have a safe labor and birth.

ADDITIONAL COMPLICATIONS

Table 2–1 describes additional complications the nurse may encounter.

Table 2–1   Selected Complications during Pregnancy

Condition/Overview	Signs/Symptoms/Risk	Medical Therapy	Nursing Interventions
Acquired Immunodeficiency Syndrome (AIDS)			
AIDS, caused by the human immunodeficiency virus (HIV), is a multisystem disorder that enters the body through blood, blood products, and body fluids such as semen, vaginal fluid, and urine. HIV affects T cells, thereby depressing the body's immune response. The highest incidence of AIDS occurs in homosexual or bisexual men, heterosexual partners of persons with AIDS, IV drug users, hemophiliacs, and fetuses of women at risk or HIV positive. Persons generally test positive for HIV within weeks to 6 months of exposure but may remain asymptomatic for 5–10 years or more.	The following women are considered at risk for AIDS: prostitutes; women with a history of sexually transmitted infection; IV drug users; and partners (currently or previously) of IV drug users, bisexual men, hemophiliacs, or those who test positive for HIV. Women with AIDS may have any of the following: malaise, weight loss, lymphadenopathy, diarrhea, fever, neurologic dysfunction, immunodeficiency, esophageal candidiasis, herpes simplex virus, vaginal *Candida* infections, and cervical disease. Maternal risks: complications such as intrapartal or postpartal hemorrhage, postpartal infection, poor wound healing, and infections of the GI tract.	Currently there is no definitive therapy for AIDS, although many drugs are available that delay the onset of symptoms. Prenatally, a triple-therapy approach is recommended. It includes ZDV plus a second nucleoside analog such as zalcitabine, didanosine, or lamivudine combined with a protease inhibitor such as indinavir, ritonavir, or saquinavir (Public Health Service Task Force, 2007). Current goal is to detect women at risk and educate the public about the spread of AIDS. All pregnant women should be offered HIV antibody testing. Women who test positive should be counseled about the implications for themselves and the fetus/newborn. They may be offered a therapeutic abortion.	1. Assess history for risk factors. 2. Provide clear information about AIDS, ZDV therapy, and the implications for the woman, her partner, and a child should the woman become pregnant. 3. Monitor asymptomatic pregnant woman for non-specific symptoms such as fever, weight loss, persistent candidiasis (vaginal yeast infection or thrush in mouth), diarrhea, cough, skin lesions.

In the United States, the vast majority of pediatric AIDS cases have resulted from perinatal transmission from mother to child.

Fetal-neonatal risks: risk of transmission from HIV-positive mother to fetus. Rate has dropped dramatically from about 25% to less than 2% due to universal HIV prenatal testing, availability of antiretroviral prophylaxis, the use of scheduled cesarean birth, and the avoidance of breastfeeding (Public Health Service Task Force, 2007).

Women who continue pregnancy need excellent prenatal care with attention to psychosocial and teaching needs.

4. Implement appropriate isolation procedures including use of disposable latex gloves when in contact with nonintact skin, mucous membranes, or body fluids (changing chux, diapers, peripads; starting IV, drawing blood); use of protective covering such as plastic apron and glasses or eye shield when contamination from splashing may occur (vaginal exam, vaginal or cesarean birth, suctioning, care of newborn before initial bath). (Consult unit procedure manual for further specifics.)

5. Provide emotional support and nonjudgmental attitude; preserve confidentiality.

(continued)

Table 2–1   Selected Complications during Pregnancy (*continued*)

Condition/Overview	Signs/Symptoms/Risk	Medical Therapy	Nursing Interventions
	Infected infant is often asymptomatic at birth; onset of symptoms usually occurs between 9 and 18 months. Facial characteristics that may indicate the newborn has been infected early in utero with HIV include microcephaly; patulous lips; prominent, boxlike forehead; increased distance between inner canthus of eyes; and flattened nasal bridge. Signs of AIDS in infants include failure to thrive, hepatosplenomegaly, interstitial lymphocytic pneumonia, recurrent infections, neurologic abnormalities, and so forth.		

Chlamydia

Sexually transmitted infection caused by *Chlamydia trachomatis*, often found in association with gonorrhea.

Women are often asymptomatic. Symptoms may include thin or purulent vaginal discharge, frequency and burning with urination, or lower abdominal pain. Infant of woman with untreated chlamydia is at risk for newborn conjunctivitis, chlamydial pneumonia, preterm birth, or fetal demise.

Currently, CDC (2006) recommends that pregnant women be treated with a single oral dose of azithromycin, which is safe and effective. Amoxicillin 3 times per day for 7 days may also be used. Doxycycline is contraindicated in pregnancy. Erythromycin eye ointment (but not silver nitrate) can prevent conjunctivitis in the newborn.

Review signs and symptoms; explain importance of taking entire dose of medication.

Gonorrhea

Sexually transmitted infection caused by *Neisseria gonorrhoeae*.

Majority of women are asymptomatic; disease often diagnosed during routine prenatal cervical culture. If symptoms are present, they may include purulent vaginal discharge, dysuria, urinary frequency, and inflammation and swelling of vulva. Cervix may appear eroded. Infection at time of birth may cause ophthalmia neonatorum in the newborn.

Pregnant women are treated with ceftriaxone or cefixime. They should not receive quinolones or tetracyclines (CDC, 2006). All sexual partners are treated.

1. Review medication purpose, side effects.
2. Explain that untreated gonorrhea may result in pelvic inflammatory disease and infertility.
3. Discuss safe sexual practices.

(continued)

Table 2–1 Selected Complications during Pregnancy (*continued*)

Condition/Overview	Signs/Symptoms/Risk	Medical Therapy	Nursing Interventions
Syphilis Sexually transmitted infection caused by the spirochete *Treponema pallidum*.	Primary stage: chancre, slight fever, malaise. Chancre lasts about 4 weeks, then disappears. Secondary stage: occurs 6 weeks to 6 months after infection. Skin eruptions (condyloma lata); also symptoms of acute arthritis, liver enlargement, iritis, chronic sore throat with hoarseness. Diagnosed by blood tests such as VDRL, rapid plasma reagent, and fluorescent treponemal antibody absorption. Dark-field exam for spirochetes may be done. May be passed transplacentally to fetus. If untreated, one of the following can occur: second-trimester abortion, stillborn infant at term, congenitally infected infant, uninfected live infant.	For syphilis less than 1 year in duration: 2.4 million units benzathine penicillin G IM. For syphilis of more than 1 year's duration or of unknown duration: 2.4 million units benzathine penicillin G once a week for 3 weeks. Sexual partners should also be screened and treated (CDC, 2006).	1. Explain the risk factors and long-term effects if syphilis is not treated. 2. Explain implications for fetus/newborn. 3. Stress importance of receiving all three doses if syphilis is greater than 1 year in duration.

Toxoplasmosis

Toxoplasmosis is caused by the protozoan *Toxoplasma gondii* and transmitted by eating raw or poorly cooked meat or by exposure to feces of infected cats. Innocuous in adults.

Toxoplasmosis results in a mild infection in adults but is associated with an increased risk of spontaneous abortion, prematurity, stillbirth, neonatal death, and disorders including microcephaly, hydrocephalus, convulsions, blindness, deafness, and mental retardation.

Goal is to identify women at risk. Diagnosis made using serologic testing, physical findings, and history. If infection is confirmed in a pregnant woman, she is treated with spiramycin. If fetal infection is suspected, spiramycin should be replaced with pyrimethamine, folinic acid, and a sulfoonamide after the 18th week of pregnancy (Duff, 2007). If toxoplasmosis is diagnosed before 20 weeks' gestation, therapeutic abortion may be offered because damage to the fetus tends to be more severe than if the disease is diagnosed later in pregnancy.

Explain methods of prevention to childbearing woman. She should avoid poorly cooked or raw meat, especially pork, beef, and lamb. Fruits and vegetables should be washed. Litter box should be cleaned frequently by someone else, and woman should wear gloves when gardening.

(continued)

The At-Risk Antepartal Client   63

Table 2–1   Selected Complications during Pregnancy (continued)

Condition/Overview	Signs/Symptoms/Risk	Medical Therapy	Nursing Interventions
Rubella			
Rubella or German measles is caused by a virus.	Rubella exposure in the first trimester is associated with spontaneous abortion, congenital heart disease, intrauterine growth restriction, cataracts, mental retardation, and cerebral palsy. Infection in the second trimester is most often associated with permanent hearing impairment in the newborn.	Best therapy is prevention by vaccination. Women of childbearing age should be tested for immunity and vaccinated if susceptible. Hemagglutination inhibition titer of 1:8 or greater indicates immunity. Pregnant women are not vaccinated but will be offered vaccination postpartum. If infection occurs in first trimester, woman will be offered a therapeutic abortion.	Assess for signs of rubella infection (maculopapular rash, lymphadenopathy, muscular achiness, joint pain). Provide emotional support and objective information for couples contemplating therapeutic abortion.
Cytomegalic Inclusion Disease (CID)			
CID is caused by the cytomegalovirus (CMV). Chronic persistent infection with viral shedding may last for years. Usually is asymptomatic in adults and children.	CID may cause fetal death; in neonates it is associated with microcephaly, cerebral palsy, mental retardation, and so forth. Subclinical infections may cause neurologic and hearing problems that may go unrecognized for months or years.	Diagnosis is confirmed by serologic tests to detect CMV antibodies. No effective treatment is available at this time.	Provide emotional support and objective information.

Herpes Simplex Virus Type 2 (HSV-2)

Genital herpes, caused by HSV-2, is a chronic recurring infection that causes painful lesions in the genital area and is transmitted by sexual contact.

Genital herpes may cause spontaneous abortion if active, primary HSV-2 infection occurs in first trimester. Highest risk of infection for newborn who is born vaginally when mother has active HSV-2 in her vagina. Risk of neonatal death, permanent brain damage, characteristic skin lesions.

Antiviral therapy may be used for women with primary HSV infection during pregnancy to decrease viral shedding and promote healing. Three medications are available: acyclovir, valaclovir, and famciclovir. Women with recurrent infection may also be treated with antiviral therapy. Vaginal birth is preferred if there is no evidence of genital infection. If there are any lesions or prodromal symptoms such as vulvar pain or burning, cesarean birth is indicated. Women with active HSV infection and ruptured membranes should give birth by cesarean as soon as possible.

Provide information about the disease and its spread. Advise woman to inform future healthcare providers of her infection. A possible association exists between herpes and cervical cancer. Thus women should understand the importance of yearly Papanicolaou smears. Provide emotional support and nonjudgmental attitude.

(continued)

Table 2–1   Selected Complications during Pregnancy *(continued)*

Condition/Overview	Signs/Symptoms/Risk	Medical Therapy	Nursing Interventions
Substance Abuse			
Indiscriminate use of alcohol or drugs such as cocaine, PCP, opiates, and methadone may affect the woman and her fetus/newborn. Alcohol abuse has been associated with fetal alcohol syndrome. Use of addicting drugs may cause the infant to be born addicted or to have serious and permanent problems.	Signs of addiction in the pregnant woman may include dilated or constricted pupils, inflamed nasal mucosa, abscesses, edema or track marks on arms and legs, inappropriate or disoriented behavior, or excessive fatigue. Risks to the fetus include the following (varies somewhat according to substance abuse): neurologic changes, including marked irritability, poor interactive behavior, poor consolability, seizures, and so forth.	Following diagnosis, management involves a team approach to provide care for woman and fetus/newborn. Hospitalization may be necessary to achieve detoxification. "Cold turkey" withdrawal is not advised because of risk to fetus. Urine screening may be done regularly throughout the pregnancy for women who are known or suspected substance abusers.	1. *Be alert for signs* of substance abuse. If it is suspected, ask direct questions, beginning with less threatening questions about use of tobacco, caffeine, and alcohol consumption. Then progress to questions about illicit drugs. 2. Provide information about the possible effects of substance abuse on the fetus.

Multiple Gestation

Morbidity and mortality rates increase significantly in pregnancies with multiple fetuses. Dizygotic, or fraternal, twins (resulting from two ova) are more common. Incidence of fraternal twins is affected by heredity, race, maternal age and parity, and fertility drugs. Monozygotic, or identical, twins (resulting from one ovum) are not as common. Incidence is not influenced by external factors other than infertility therapy. Higher numbers of fetuses (triplets or quadruplets, for example) may result from infertility therapy.

Fetal risk is significantly higher. The perinatal mortality rate is higher, and there is an increased risk of preterm labor with the problems associated with prematurity. Multiple gestation increases the incidence of intrauterine growth restriction (IUGR), congenital anomalies, and abnormal presentations. For the mother, a multiple gestation may contribute to more physical discomfort during pregnancy, such as shortness of breath, backaches, and pedal edema as well as an increased incidence of preeclampsia, anemia, and placenta previa. Prolonged hospitalization may be necessary, especially with three or more fetuses.

Preventing preterm labor is a major goal. Early diagnosis is based on history and greater-than-anticipated uterine size. Ultrasound is crucial. Women are seen every 2 weeks until 28 weeks' gestation and then weekly. Serial ultrasounds are done regularly to assess for IUGR; NST and fetal biophysical profile are done at least weekly beginning at 28–30 weeks. Bed rest in the lateral position may be suggested as early as 23–26 weeks to prevent preterm labor. Maternal blood pressure is monitored closely. Preterm labor is managed in the same way as it is for single pregnancy (see earlier discussion in this chapter).

1. Counsel on importance of good nutrition, including adequate calories (at least 3,500 kcal) and 175 g protein. A prenatal vitamin with iron and 1 mg folic acid should be taken daily (Newman & Rittenberg, 2008).

2. Discuss importance of sufficient rest if at home (usually bed rest with BRP) or at least 2 hours in the morning, afternoon, and evening.

3. If woman is hospitalized, explain importance of complete bed rest (or bed rest with BRP if ordered).

(continued)

Table 2–1   Selected Complications during Pregnancy (*continued*)

Condition/Overview	Signs/Symptoms/Risk	Medical Therapy	Nursing Interventions
			4. Monitor fetal status. This involves isolating each FHR as well as running an electronic fetal monitor strip on each fetus at least q4–8h (depending on agency policy). If possible, run the strips at the same time, using two (or three) monitors. This becomes more difficult with quadruplets.
			5. Monitor for signs of complications such as preeclampsia or preterm labor.

BRP, bathroom privileges; CDC, Centers for Disease Control and Prevention; FHR, fetal heart rate; GI, gastrointestinal; IM, intramuscularly; IV, intravenously; NST, nonstress test; PCP, phencyclidine; ZDV, zidovudine.

REFERENCES

American College of Obstetricians and Gynecologists (ACOG). (2000). *Scheduled cesarean delivery and the prevention of the vertical transmission of HIV infection* (ACOG Committee Opinion No. 234). Washington, DC: Author.

American College of Obstetricians and Gynecologists (ACOG). (2005). *Pregestational diabetes mellitus* (ACOG Practice Bulletin No. 60). Washington, DC: Author.

American Diabetes Association. (2006). Position statement: Gestational diabetes mellitus. *Diabetes Care, 29*(Suppl 1).

Carey, J. C., & Gibbs, R. S. (2008). Preterm labor and posterm delivery. In R. S. Gibbs, B. Y. Karlan, A. F. Haney, & I. E. Nygaard (Eds.), *Danforth's obstetrics and gynecology* (10th ed.). Philadelphia: Wolters Kluwer/Lippincott Williams & Wilkins.

Centers for Disease Control and Prevention (CDC). (2006, August 4). Sexually transmitted disease guidelines, 2006. *Morbidity and Mortality Weekly Report, 55*(RR-11), 1–93.

Cleveland Clinic. (2006). Gestational diabetes. Hypoglycemia. Retrieved July 7, 2007, from http://www.clevelandclinic.org/health/health-info/docs/2300/2354.asp?index=9012.

Duff, P. (2007). Maternal and perinatal infection—bacterial. In S. G. Gabbe, J. R. Niebyl, & J. L. Simpson (Eds.), *Obstetrics: Normal and problem pregnancies* (5th ed.). Philadelphia: Churchill Livingstone.

Fowles, E. R. (2004). Clinical issues. Prenatal nutrition and birth outcomes. *JOGNN: Journal of Obstetric, Gynecologic, and Neonatal Nursing, 33*(6), 809–822.

Iams, J. D., & Romero, R. (2007). Preterm birth. In S. G. Gabbe, J. R. Niebyl, & J. L. Simpson (Eds.), *Obstetrics: Normal and problem pregnancies* (5th ed.). Philadelphia: Churchill Livingstone.

Ness, A., Visintine, J., Ricci, E., & Berghella, V. (2007). Does knowledge of cervical length and fetal fibronectin affect management of women with threatened preterm labor? A randomized trial. *American Journal of Obstetricians & Gynecologists, 197*(4), 426.e1–7.

Newman, R. B., & Rittenberg, C. (2008). Multiple gestation. In R. S. Gibbs, B. Y. Karlan, A. F. Haney, & I. E. Nygaard (Eds.), *Danforth's obstetrics and gynecology* (10th ed.). Philadelphia: Wolters Kluwer/Lippincott Williams & Wilkins.

Newton, E. R. (2005). Preterm labor, preterm premature rupture of membranes, and chorioamnionitis. *Clinics in Perinatology, 32,* 571–600.

Perkins, J. M., Dunn, J. P., & Jagasia, S. (2007). Perspectives in gestational diabetes mellitus: A review of screening, diagnosis, and treatment. *Clinical Diabetes, 25*(2), 57–62.

Public Health Service Task Force. (2007, November 2). Recommendations for use of antiretroviral drugs in pregnant HIV-infected women for maternal health and interventions to reduce perinatal HIV-1 transmission in the United States. Retrieved May 19, 2008, from http://aidsinfo.nih.gov.

Reece, E. A., & Homko, C. J. (2008). Diabetes mellitus and pregnancy. In R. S. Gibbs, B. Y. Karlan, A. F. Haney, & I. E. Nygaard (Eds.), *Danforth's obstetrics and gynecology* (10th ed.). Philadelphia: Wolters Kluwer/Lippincott Williams & Wilkins.

Sabai, B. M. (2007). Hypertension. In S. G. Gabbe, J. R. Niebyl, & J. L. Simpson (Eds.), *Obstetrics: Normal and problem pregnancies* (5th ed.). Philadelphia: Churchill Livingstone.

Tekesin, I., Marek, S., Hellmeyer, L., Reits, D., & Schmidt, S. (2005). Assessment of rapid fetal fibronectin in predicting preterm delivery. *Obstetrics & Gynecology, 105*(2), 280–284.

3 THE INTRAPARTAL CLIENT

Labor and birth progresses through four stages. A first-time laboring woman (nullipara) averages 13 hours (11 hours in first stage and 2 hours of pushing in second stage). A multipara averages about 8 hours (7¼ hours in first stage and 1 hour pushing in second stage). See Table 3–1 for definitions of each stage of labor.

NURSING CARE DURING ADMISSION

Admission is a critical time for data collection that will aid in the formation of nursing care for the laboring family.

* Orient laboring woman and her support team to the room and the equipment.
* Instruct woman to change into hospital gown.
* Obtain a urine specimen if membranes are intact and woman is not bleeding.
* Assess uterine activity, fetal status, and status of membranes.
* Assess temperature, blood pressure, pulse, respirations, and pain level.
* Complete admission forms and consent forms.
* Review prenatal record for history of pregnancy (present and past), preexisting medical problems, estimated date of birth (EDB), risk factors, blood type and Rh, allergies, medications, and history of psychologic disorders or substance abuse. If the woman has had a previous cesarean birth, documentation of the previous uterine incision is needed.
* Discuss the method of desired pain management.
* Determine the desired role of the support team.

3

Table 3–1   Stages of Labor and Birth

Stage	Begins	Ends
First	Beginning of cervical dilatation	Complete dilatation
Second	Complete dilatation	Birth of the baby
Third	Birth of the baby	Birth of the placenta
Fourth	Birth of the placenta	1–4 hours past birth

- Notify physician or certified nurse-midwife (CNM) of woman's labor status.
- See Table 3–2 for deviations from normal labor process that require immediate interventions.

Sample Admission Nurse's Charting

Grav I Para 0 EDB 7/13. 40 wks gestation. Admitted ambulatory to BR1 in labor. Contractions q3min, 50 sec duration of mod. quality. Membranes intact. Cervix 5 cm, 80% effaced, soft and anterior. Small amount blood-tinged mucus present. Vertex presentation at 0 station. FHR 140 by external fetal monitoring. No increase or decrease in FHR noted during or following UC. Marked variability. NST reactive. Maternal temp 98.6°F, pulse 78, resp 18 BP 120/74. Pt states pain is a 5 on a scale of 1–10 (10 being the most intense pain). Admission UA obtained and to lab. Support person with pt and to remain through birth. Pt oriented to room. P. Gomez, RNC

ASSESSMENT OF UTERINE ACTIVITY DURING LABOR

- Uterine activity can be assessed by either palpation or electronic monitoring.
- Assess for frequency, duration, and intensity. (*Note:* Assess a minimum of three consecutive contractions when evaluating uterine activity.)
- See Table 3–3 for contraction and labor progress characteristics.
  1. **Frequency** is timed from the beginning of a contraction (when the uterus first begins to tighten) to the beginning of the next contraction. Frequency is recorded in half- or full-minute increments (1½–3 minutes).

Table 3-2 Deviations from Normal Labor Process Requiring Immediate Intervention

Finding	Immediate Action	Finding	Immediate Action
Woman admitted with unusual vaginal bleeding or history of painless vaginal bleeding	1. Do not perform vaginal examination. 2. Assess and continually monitor FHR. 3. Evaluate amount of blood loss. 4. Evaluate labor pattern. 5. Notify physician/CNM immediately.	Prolapse of umbilical cord	1. Relieve pressure on cord manually by holding up the presenting part. 2. Continuously monitor FHR; watch for changes in FHR pattern. 3. Notify physician/CNM. 4. Assist woman into knee-chest position. 5. Administer oxygen. 6. Direct another person to prepare for immediate cesarean section. 7. Watch for decreasing baseline, loss of variability, presence of late or variable decelerations.

(continued)

Table 3-2 Deviations from Normal Labor Process Requiring Immediate Intervention (*continued*)

Finding	Immediate Action	Finding	Immediate Action
Presence of greenish or brownish amniotic fluid	1. Continuously monitor FHR. 2. Evaluate dilatation status of cervix and determine whether umbilical cord is prolapsed. 3. Evaluate presentation (vertex or breech). 4. Maintain woman on complete bed rest on left side. 5. Notify physician/CNM immediately. 6. Note color and consistency of amniotic fluid.		

Absence of FHR and fetal movement	1. Notify physician/CNM. 2. Provide truthful information and emotional support to laboring couple. 3. Remain with the couple. 4. Prepare for diagnostic ultrasound exam.	

	Woman admitted in advanced labor; birth imminent	1. Prepare for immediate birth.
		2. Obtain critical information:
		  a. EDB
		  b. History of bleeding problems
		  c. Identifying absence of placenta previa
		  d. History of medical or obstetrical problems
		  e. Past and or present use/abuse of prescription/OTC/illicit drugs
		  f. Problems with this pregnancy
		  g. FHR and maternal vital signs if possible
		  h. Whether membranes are ruptured and how long since rupture
		  i. Blood type and Rh
		3. Direct another person to contact CNM/physician; do not leave woman alone.
		4. Provide support to couple.
		5. Put on gloves.

CNM, certified nurse-midwife; EDB, estimated date of birth; FHR, fetal heart rate; OTC, over the counter.

Table 3-3   Contraction and Labor Progress Characteristics

Contraction Characteristics	
Latent Phase	Every 10–30 min × 30 sec; mild, progressing to Every 5–7 min × 30–40 sec; moderate
Active phase	Every 2–5 min × 40–60 sec; moderate to strong
Transition phase	Every 1½–2 min × 60–90 sec; strong
Labor Progress Characteristics	
Primipara	At least 1.2 cm/hr dilatation
	At least 1 cm/hr descent
	Less than 2 h in second stage (3 hr with epidural)
Multipara	At least 1.5 cm/hr dilatation
	At least 2 cm/h descent
	Less than 1 hr in second stage (2 h with epidural)

2. **Duration** is timed from the beginning of a contraction (when the uterus first begins to tighten) to the end of that same contraction (when the uterus fully relaxes). Duration is recorded in seconds (30–90 seconds).

3. **Intensity** refers to the strength of a contraction during the acme. It is evaluated by estimating the indentability of the fundus at the acme of the contraction when using palpation as method of evaluation or by the use of an intrauterine pressure catheter (IUPC). Intensity is recorded as mild, moderate, or strong when palpating contraction and in millimeters of mercury when using an IUPC.

- See Figure 3–1 for characteristics of uterine contractions.

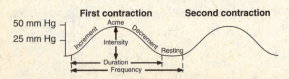

Figure 3–1 ■ Characteristics of uterine contractions.

Palpating Uterine Contractions

- With the woman's gown over her abdomen but blanket pulled down, place palmar surface of fingertips on the fundal area of the uterus.
- Assess for frequency, duration, and intensity.
  1. Mild intensity: At the acme of the contraction, the fingertips can easily indent the abdomen.
  2. Moderate intensity: At the acme of the contraction, the fingertips can slightly indent the abdomen.
  3. Strong: At the acme of the contraction, the fingertips cannot indent the abdomen.
- Record assessment findings in chart.

Assessment of Uterine Activity by External Electronic Uterine Monitoring

- With the woman's gown up and blanket down, place the tocodynamometer against the fundal area of the uterus. The tocodynamometer is held in place with elastic belts.
- Assess for frequency and duration.
- Uterine contraction intensity cannot be evaluated accurately with external electronic monitoring. Manual palpation is needed to assess uterine contraction intensity.
- Record assessment findings in chart.

Assessment by Intrauterine Pressure Catheter (IUPC)

- Membranes must be ruptured before placement of the IUPC.
- The prenatal ultrasound report should be reviewed to assess for placenta location before the insertion of an IUPC.
- Explain procedure to woman and her labor support team.
- Have IUPC in room ready for placement.
- CNM or physician inserts IUPC into uterine cavity.

- IUPC is connected to electronic monitor.
- Frequency, duration, and intensity are recorded on the monitor strip.
- Normal resting pressure is below 20 mm Hg.
- During the acme the intensity ranges from:
  1. 25–40 mm Hg in the latent phase
  2. 50–70 mm Hg in the active phase
  3. 70–90 mm Hg in the transition phase
  4. 70–100 mm Hg in the second stage while the woman is pushing

Frequency of Assessments for Low-Risk Mother

- First stage: every 30 minutes
- Second stage: every 15 minutes

Frequency of Assessments for High-Risk Mother

- First stage: every 15 minutes
- Second stage: every 5 minutes

Assessment of Cervical Changes

Cervical assessment evaluates cervical dilatation and effacement as well as position and consistency of the cervix. These data are obtained by intrapartal vaginal examination (Figure 3–2). See Procedures: Performing an Intrapartal Vaginal Examination, pp. 338–342.

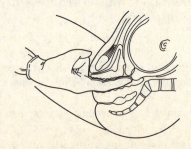

Figure 3–2 ■ Determination of cervical dilatation.

Dilatation: Enlargement of the external cervical os from 0–10 cm.

Effacement: The drawing up of the internal os and cervical canal into the uterine side wall. This is measured in percentages: 0% indicates no effacement and 100% indicates full effacement. In nulliparas, effacement usually precedes dilatation.

Position: The position of the cervix in the vagina. This is described as posterior, midposition, or anterior. A posterior cervix is far back in the vagina and requires the examiner to reach far back into the vagina to locate it. An anterior cervix is located closer to the opening of the vagina and does not require the examiner to reach as far back. A midposition cervix is halfway between a posterior and anterior position.

Consistency: The consistency of the cervix is described as firm, medium, or soft.

ASSESSMENT OF AMNIOTIC FLUID MEMBRANES

It is important to determine whether amniotic membranes are intact or ruptured. The woman's risk for ascending bacterial infection is increased after the membranes have ruptured. The degree of risk increases as the length of time past rupture increases.

Membranes Ruptured before Admission to Labor Unit

- Ask woman when the membranes ruptured (when she felt a gush of fluid from her vagina).
- Note the color (should be colorless), odor (should be odorless), and amount (small, moderate, or large) of fluid.
- To confirm the rupture of membranes, the nurse can check with Nitrazine paper, or a fern test can be performed.
- **Nitrazine paper test**
  1. Explain procedure to woman, and position for intrapartal exam.

2. Items needed: sterile glove and Nitrazine paper.
3. With a sterile, unlubricated, gloved hand, insert Nitrazine into cervical area and remove it.
4. Nitrazine paper is sensitive to pH and will turn blue when exposed to amniotic fluid.
5. Discuss findings with woman.

- **Fern test**
  1. Explain procedure to woman, and position for intrapartal exam.
  2. Items needed: sterile glove(s), Q-Tip, and slide.
  3. With a sterile gloved hand, obtain a swabbed specimen of vaginal fluid.
  4. Apply fluid to a microscopic slide, and let dry. Then observe slide under magnification.
  5. A fern-like pattern will appear with crystallization of amniotic fluid.
  6. Discuss findings with woman.
- Assess fetal status via auscultation or electronic fetal monitoring (see Assessment of Fetus).
- Assess for prolapsed cord via intrapartal exam.
- Chart findings, including date and time of rupture, color of fluid, odor of fluid, amount of fluid, and fetal status.

Membranes Rupture after Admission to Labor Unit

- Note the time of rupture, the color of the fluid, the odor, and the amount.
- Assess fetal heart rate (FHR) via auscultation or electronic fetal monitoring.
- There is an increased risk of a prolapsed umbilical cord if the membranes rupture before engagement of the presenting part. Assess for prolapsed cord via intrapartal exam: Can you feel the cord around the cervical area?
- Chart findings that include time of rupture, color of fluid, odor of fluid, amount of fluid, and fetal status.

ASSESSMENT OF FETUS
Fetal Heart Rate
FHR can be assessed with the use of a fetoscope, Doppler, tocotransducer, or fetal scalp electrode.

- **Baseline rate:** Refers to the range of FHR observed between contractions during a 10-minute period of monitoring. The range does not include the rate present during decelerations. Normal range is 110–160 beats per minute.
- **Baseline changes:** Defined in terms of 10-minute periods of time. Changes include tachycardia, bradycardia, and variability of heart rate.
- **Tachycardia:** FHR above 160 beats per minute continuing for 10 minutes or longer.
- **Bradycardia:** FHR less than 110 beats per minute continuing for 10 minutes or longer.
- **Periodic changes:** Refers to the presence of acceleration and deceleration.
- Other characteristics of electronic fetal monitoring (EFM) tracings are presented in Table 3–4.

Assessment Using Fetoscope or Doppler
See Procedures: Auscultation of Fetal Heart Rate, pp. 324–325.

Assessment Using External Electronic Fetal Monitor
See Procedures: Electronic Fetal Monitoring, pp. 325–327.

Evaluation of Fetal Monitor Tracing
Evaluation of monitor tracing includes uterine activity and FHR. A 10-minute strip is needed to evaluate uterine activity and FHR. See Figure 3–3.

- Uterine activity
  1. Determine uterine resting tone.
  2. Determine frequency, duration, and intensity of the contractions.
- FHR
  1. Determine baseline rate.
  2. Assess for bradycardia or tachycardia.
  3. Determine if FHR is reactive or nonreactive.

Table 3–4   Characteristics of Fetal Heart Rate (FHR) Tracings

Example	Characteristic	Nursing Intervention
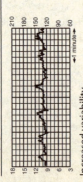 Increased variability	*Variability* Caused by interplay of sympathetic and parasympathetic nervous systems. Variability classification: Decreased/minimal: 0–5 beats per minute Moderate/average: 6–25 beats per minute Marked (saltatory): Greater than 25 beats per minute	Maximize uteroplacental perfusion by positioning woman on left side. Document findings; report status to certified nurse-midwife (CNM) or physician. Correct maternal hypotension by turning woman to side-lying position, increasing rate of intravenous infusion.
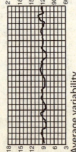 Average variability	*Nonperiodic Accelerations* An increase of FHR that lasts for a few seconds. Occurs with fetal movement. Is basis of nonstress test (NST).	For the most part, there are no specific interventions.
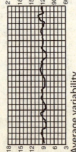 Absent variability		

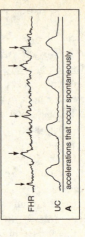

FHR

UC

A accelerations that occur spontaneously

Deceleration

Periodic decrease in FHR from the normal baseline.

Classified as early, late, or variable.

Early Deceleration (Periodic)

Due to pressure on the fetal head as it progresses down the birth canal.

Characteristics:

Resembles upside-down shape of uterine contraction.

Occurs at or just before the beginning of contraction and ends as contraction ends.

Nadir (lowest point) occurs at peak of contraction and is within normal FHR range.

Is considered a normal variation.

No specific intervention needed.

Monitor for changes in FHR pattern.

Evaluate for possible cephalopelvic disproportion (CPD) if occurs in early labor.

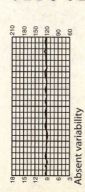

Absent variability

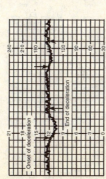

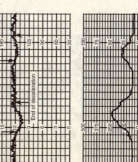

Early deceleration

(continued)

Table 3–4   Characteristics of Fetal Heart Rate (FHR) Tracings (continued)

Example	Characteristic	Nursing Intervention
	Late Deceleration (Periodic) Due to uteroplacental insufficiency as the result of decreased blood flow and oxygen transfer to the fetus during contractions.	Turn woman to left side-lying position. Report findings to physician/CNM and document findings. Provide explanation to woman and partner.
	Characteristics:	Monitor for further FHR changes.
	Smooth, uniform shape that inversely mirrors contraction.	Maintain good hydration with IV fluids. Discontinue oxytocin if it is being administered.
	Begins at or within seconds after the peak of the contraction.	Administer oxygen by face mask at 7–10 L/min.
	Lasts past end of contraction.	Monitor maternal BP, P for signs of hypotension.
	Tends to occur with every contraction; persistent and consistent.	Assist with preparation for cesarean birth if required.
Late decelerations	Usually occurs within normal FHR range.	
	In some situations, changing maternal position, providing IV hydration, and decreasing contraction frequency will decrease late decelerations.	

Variable Deceleration

Due to umbilical cord compression, which decreases the amount of blood flow (therefore oxygen supply) to the fetus.

Characteristics:

Varies in onset, occurrence, and waveform.

Usually falls outside the normal FHR range.

Is acute in onset.

Document findings.

Report status to CNM/physician.

Change maternal position to one on which FHR pattern is most improved.

Provide explanation to woman and partner.

Discontinue oxytocin if it is being administered and there are severe variables.

Oxytocin may be continued if mild or moderate decelerations are present.

Perform vaginal examination to assess for prolapsed cord or change in labor progress.

Monitor FHR continuously to assess current status and for further changes in FHR pattern.

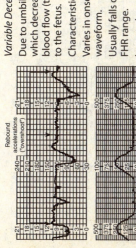

Variable decelerations

BP, blood pressure; IV, intravenous; P, pulse; UC, uterine contraction.

Source: Association of Women's Health, Obstetrical, and Neonatal Nurses (AWHONN), 1997.

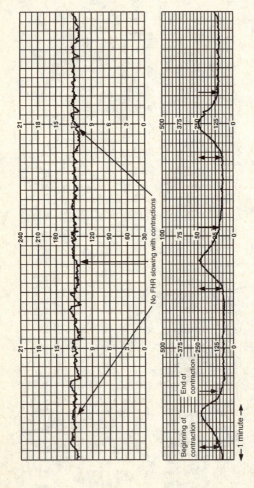

Figure 3–3 ■ Normal fetal heart rate (FHR) range is from 110–160 beats per minute. The FHR tracing in the upper portion of the graph indicates FHR range of 140–155 beats per minute. The lower portion is a tracing of the uterine contraction pattern (frequency and duration of contractions).

- Determine variability: Is it marked, average, minimal, or absent? Assess for accelerations, decelerations, and sinusoidal pattern.
- Assess for periodic changes (see Types of Periodic Changes section).
- See Table 3–4 for characteristics of FHR tracings.

Types of Periodic Changes

- **Accelerations:** Transient increases in FHR of 15 beats per minute above baseline for 15 seconds. They are usually caused by fetal movement. These are signs of fetal well-being.
- **Early decelerations:** Decelerations that begin with the onset of a contraction and end before the contraction ends. They are uniform in shape and are due to fetal head compression. Interventions are not needed.
- **Late decelerations:** Decelerations that start after the beginning of the contraction and end after the contraction ends. They are uniform in shape and are due to uteroplacental insufficiency. Interventions are needed.
- **Variable decelerations:** Decelerations that vary in onset, occurrence, and shape. They are due to umbilical cord compression. Interventions are needed.

Classifying the Fetal Heart Rate Tracing as Reassuring or Nonreassuring

- Reassuring pattern: FHR baseline between 110 and 160 beats per minute, variability present, acceleration with fetal movement, absence of late or variable deceleration.
- Nonreassuring pattern: Late decelerations, absent variability, prolonged deceleration, bradycardia, variable decelerations associated with a decrease in variability, or variable decelerations with slow return of FHR to baseline.

Note: Nonreassuring pattern may indicate nonreassuring fetal status, which requires interventions.

FETAL PRESENTATION, POSITION, AND STATION

- See Figure 3–4.
- Fetal presentation, position, and station are determined by intrapartal vaginal examination.
- *Presentation:* Refers to the part of the fetus that enters the pelvic passage first. Fetal presentation may be cephalic, breech, or transverse.
- *Position:* Refers to the relationship of a designated landmark on the presenting fetal part to the front, back, or side of the maternal pelvis. Examples of cephalic positions are the following:
  1. OA, occiput anterior
  2. ROA, right occiput anterior
  3. LOA, left occiput anterior

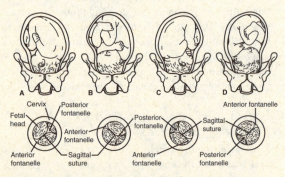

Figure 3–4 ■ Assessment of fetal position. **A,** Left occiput anterior (LOA). The posterior fontanelle (triangle shaped) is in the upper left quadrant of the maternal pelvis. **B,** Left occiput posterior (LOP). The posterior fontanelle is in the lower left quadrant of the maternal pelvis. **C,** Right occiput anterior (ROA). The posterior fontanelle is in the upper right quadrant of the maternal pelvis. **D,** Right occiput posterior (ROP). The posterior fontanelle is in the lower right quadrant of the maternal pelvis.

4. LOT, left occiput transverse
5. OP, occiput posterior
6. LOP, left occiput posterior
7. ROP, right occiput posterior

- *Station:* Refers to the relationship of the presenting part to the ischial spines. It measures fetal descent.

PSYCHOSOCIAL CONSIDERATIONS

Assessment of the woman's emotional state, her coping methods, and her support system will provide useful information for the admission process and later in the labor. Psychologic disorders can directly affect her labor experience.

- Assessment data
  1. Determine type of prenatal education program the woman has completed.
  2. Determine her hopes or plans for the labor and birth experience.
  3. Determine plans she has made with her CNM or physician.
  4. Determine her informational needs.
  5. Determine the roles of her support team.
  6. Assess for evidence of support between the woman and her partner and/or support team.
  7. Assess her past labor and birth experiences.
  8. Assess for cultural needs during labor and birth.
  9. Determine her desired method of pain management.

Assessing for Safety and Abuse Issues

- Physical and/or emotional abuse affects 15%–25% of pregnant women (Pan American Health Organization, 2006).
- Interview woman alone when assessing safety and abuse issues to ensure that she can freely answer questions.

- Questions to ask include the following:
  1. Have you ever been emotionally or physically abused by your partner or someone important to you?
  2. Within the last year, have you been hit, slapped, kicked, or otherwise physically hurt by someone? If yes, by whom? Total number of times?
  3. Since you've been pregnant, were you hit, slapped, kicked, or otherwise physically hurt by someone? If yes, by whom? Total number of times?
  4. Within the last year has anyone forced you to engage in sexual activities? If yes, who? Total number of times?
  5. Are you afraid of your partner or anyone you mentioned earlier?

CRITICAL NURSING ASSESSMENTS DURING LABOR

During the first stage of labor the nurse assesses:
- Uterine contractions
- Fetal status
- Status of membranes and amniotic fluid
- Maternal temperature, blood pressure, pulse, and respirations, and pain level
- Maternal comfort level and need for pain management assistance
- Needs for support team
- Presence of any physical or learning disabilities that will affect the woman's abilities during the first stage of labor

See Table 3–5 for nursing assessment during labor and birth.

CRITICAL NURSING INTERVENTIONS DURING LABOR

During labor, the nursing support measures vary depending on the progress of labor and the wishes of the laboring woman or couple. Table 3–6 summarizes the major

Table 3–5 Nursing Assessments in the First Stage

Phase	Mother	Fetus
First stage	Blood pressure, respirations every 30 minutes if in normal range	FHR every 30 minutes for low-risk women and every 15 minutes for high-risk women if normal characteristics present (average variability, baseline in the 110–160 beats per minute range, without late or variable decelerations).
	Temperature every 4 hours unless over 37.5°C (99.6°F) or membranes ruptured, then every hour	
	Uterine contractions every 30 minutes	Note fetal activity.
		If electronic fetal monitor in place, assess for reactive NST.
Second stage	Blood pressure, pulse, respirations every 15 minutes	FHR every 15 minutes if normal characteristics are present. In high-risk women, assess every 5 minutes.
	Contractions palpated at least every 15 minutes	

FHR, fetal heart rate; NST, nonstress test.
Source: American College of Obstetrics & Gynecology (ACOG), 2005.

characteristics of labor and birth and presents nursing interventions that may be used in each stage of labor.

NONPHARMACOLOGIC PAIN MANAGEMENT DURING LABOR

- Pain during the first stage of labor is due to cervical stretching.
- Pain during the second stage of labor is due to stretching of the vagina and perineum.
- A variety of methods and techniques can be used for labor pain management.
- Nonpharmacologic methods include visualization, relaxation techniques, breathing patterns, acupressure, acupuncture, meditation, massage, and touch.

Visualization Method

- Direct the woman to visualize a place where she has a pleasant memory or feeling: "Think of a place where you have been that has pleasant memories and feelings

Table 3–6 Normal Progress, Psychologic Characteristics, and Nursing Support during First and Second Stages of Labor

Stage/Phase	Cervical Dilatation	Uterine Contractions	Woman's Response	Nursing Support Measures
Stage 1 Latent phase	1–3 cm	Every 10–30 min; 30 sec duration; mild intensity progressing to moderate.	Usually happy, talkative, and eager to be in labor. Exhibits need for independence by taking care of own bodily needs and seeking information.	Establish rapport on admission and continue to build during care. Assess information base and learning needs. Be available to consult regarding breathing technique if needed; teach breathing technique if needed and in early labor. Orient family to room, equipment, monitors, and procedures. Encourage woman and partner to participate in care as desired. Provide needed information. Assist woman into position of comfort (nonsupine position); encourage frequent change of position; and encourage ambulation during early labor. Offer fluids/ice chips. Keep couple informed of progress. Encourage woman to void every 1–2 hours. Assess need for and interest in using visualization to enhance relaxation, and teach if appropriate.

| Active phase | 4–7 cm | Every 2–5 min; 40–60 sec duration; moderate to strong intensity. | May experience feelings of helplessness; exhibits increased fatigue and may begin to feel restless and anxious or frustrated as contractions become stronger; expresses fear of abandonment. Becomes more dependent as she is less able to meet her needs. | Observe response to contractions. Encourage woman to maintain breathing patterns; provide quiet environment to reduce external stimuli. Provide reassurance, encouragement, support; keep couple informed of progress. Promote comfort by giving back rubs, sacral pressure, cool cloth on forehead, suggest position changes and other comfort measures, support with pillows, effleurage. Provide ice chips, ointment for dry mouth and lips. Encourage to void every 1–2 hours. Offer shower/Jacuzzi/warm bath if available. |

(continued)

Table 3–6 Normal Progress, Psychologic Characteristics, and Nursing Support during First and Second Stages of Labor (continued)

Stage/Phase	Cervical Dilatation	Uterine Contractions	Woman's Response	Nursing Support Measures
Transition	8–10 cm	Every 1½–2 min; 60–90 sec duration; strong intensity.	Tires and may exhibit increased restlessness and irritability; may feel she cannot keep up with labor process and is out of control. Physical discomforts. Fear of being left alone. May fear tearing open or splitting apart with contractions.	Encourage woman to rest between contractions; if she sleeps between contractions, wake her at beginning of contraction so she can begin breathing pattern (increases feeling of control). Provide support, encouragement, and praise for efforts. Keep couple informed of progress; encourage continued participation of support persons. Promote comfort as noted earlier, but recognize that many women do not want to be touched when in transition. Provide privacy. Provide ice chips, ointment for lips. Encourage to void every 1–2 hours. If she has difficulty focusing, cup your hands close to her face and place your face close to hers. Talk her through the contraction. Have her breathe with you. Stay with her.

| Stage 2 | Complete | Every 2 min; 60–90 sec duration; strong intensity. | May feel out of control, helpless, panicky, exhausted, exhilarated. | Assist woman in pushing efforts. Encourage woman to assume position of comfort. She may be most comfortable in a sitting position on a toilet, leaning over a birthing bar, on hands and knees, or perhaps on her side. Some women like to sit in high Fowler's, to have support behind their shoulders, and to have someone hold their legs up and flexed while they push. Provide encouragement and praise for efforts. Keep couple informed of progress. Provide ice chips and cool cloth for forehead. Many women feel hot at this stage. Fanning with a glove package can provide relief if a fan is not available. Maintain privacy as woman desires. |

around it, a place that was relaxing, where all your stress disappeared."

- Ask the woman to take in a breath and remember the smells around the place. If it was outside, instruct her to feel the warmth of the sun or the way the breeze felt on her face.
- Instruct her to mentally sit in that place again and let all her tension and tiredness leave her body as she feels the warmth and breezes.
- Give the woman a few moments to think about her special place. Ask if she would like to share information about the setting.
- After the woman has a visualization set up, suggest thinking about it during contractions as a means of increasing relaxation and focusing concentration.
- As each contraction begins, instruct her to think about this special place for a moment and let her body relax.
- Instruct her to keep a picture of her place in her mind as she breathes with the contraction.
- When the contraction is over, instruct her to let her body stay relaxed and to feel the comfort of the room and support of those around her.

Relaxation Techniques

- Assist the woman into a comfortable position (mid-Fowler's with arms supported by pillows, or side-lying with pillow between knees and pillows to support arms, or in a reclining or rocking chair).
- Teach her to breathe slowly and easily and to close her eyes and to let her body sink into the bed (or chair).
- Adjust her position so that each part of her body is supported and comfortable.
- Instruct her to maintain her breathing and try to keep her mind clear.
- Assist her to focus by instructing her to think of the number 1 as she inhales, and the number 2 as she exhales.
- Explain to her that each time her mind begins to drift away to quietly think about the numbers.

- Recommend that she tighten her face, hold it a few seconds, and then release all the tightness. Encourage her to let her tension flow out with her breath.
- A variation of this exercise is to have the woman tighten a body part, hold for a few seconds, and then release it as the coach lightly strokes that body part. Later in labor, gentle stroking of the woman's arms or back will enhance relaxation.

Lamaze Breathing Patterns

- Slow-paced breathing pattern
  1. This pattern begins and ends with a cleansing breath.
  2. Cleansing breath is inhaled through the nose and exhaled through pursed lips as if cooling a spoonful of hot food.
  3. While inhaling through the nose and exhaling through pursed lips, slow breaths are taken, moving only the chest.
  4. The rate should be approximately 6–9 per minute or 2 breaths in 15 seconds.
  5. The coach or nurse may assist by reminding the woman to take a cleansing breath, and then the coach or nurse could count out the breaths if needed to maintain pacing.
  6. The woman inhales as someone counts "one one thousand, two one thousand, three one thousand, four one thousand." Exhalation begins and continues through the same count.
- Modified-paced breathing pattern
  1. This pattern begins and ends with a cleansing breath.
  2. Breaths are then taken in and out silently through the mouth at approximately 4 breaths in 5 seconds.
  3. The jaw and entire body need to be relaxed.
  4. The rate can be accelerated to 2–2½ breaths per second.
  5. The rhythm for the breaths can be counted out as "one and two and one and two and" with the woman exhaling on the numbers and inhaling on "and."

- Paced breathing pattern
  1. This pattern begins and ends with a cleansing breath.
  2. All breaths are rhythmical, in and out through the mouth.
  3. Exhalations are accompanied by a "Hee" or "Hoo" sound in a varying pattern, which begins as 3:1 (Hee Hee Hee Hoo) and can change to 2:1 (Hee Hee Hoo) or 1:1 (Hee Hoo) as the intensity of the contraction changes.
  4. The rate should not be more rapid than 2–2½ per second.
  5. The rhythm of the breaths would match a "one and two and" count.

Therapeutic Touch

- Some women find comfort in being touched during labor.
- Determine if the woman likes being touched.
- Touch or massage a body area of the woman such as the shoulders, arms, hands, legs, feet, or abdomen.
- The touch should be gentle and the massage should be slow and rhythmical.
- Counter sacral pressure or massage may be helpful in reducing back discomfort.

ANALGESIC AGENTS FOR USE DURING LABOR

- A variety of analgesic agents, such as butorphanol tartrate (Stadol), meperidine (Demerol), or nalbuphine hydrochloride (Nubain) (see Drug Guide), can be used for labor pain management.
- Analgesics are not given if maternal vital signs are unstable, if the woman is hypotensive, if severe hemorrhage is present, if the baby is preterm, or if the FHR is nonreassuring.

- The guidelines for administration are as follows:
  1. Assess woman and her record for history of allergies.
  2. Assess baseline FHR and maternal vital signs before administration of analgesic in order to have a comparison if hypotension or FHR changes occur. Record findings on the chart and on EFM strip (if running).
  3. Encourage woman to empty her bladder before administration of analgesic to enhance the rest and relaxation from the drug.
  4. Raise side rails to provide safety and explain this precaution to client.
  5. Monitor maternal vital signs and continuously monitor the FHR to ensure they remain in a normal range.
  6. Chart analgesic administration and maternal-fetal status on client record and on EFM tracing.

Regional Blocks
- Regional blocks include epidural, spinal-epidural, pudendal, and local infiltration.
- See Table 3–7, which highlights nursing actions during regional blocks.

Continuous Epidural Infusion
Increasing numbers of women are choosing epidurals as their method of labor pain management.
- An epidural relieves pain associated with the first stage by blocking the sensory nerve supply to the uterus.
- An epidural can also relieve pain associated with the second stage of labor.
- Nursing care for women choosing epidurals includes the following:
  1. Explain procedure and equipment, risks, and expected outcomes.

Table 3–7 Summary of Commonly Used Regional Blocks

Type of Block	Area Affected	Use during Labor and Birth	Nursing Actions
Epidural	Vagina, perineum, and uterus	Given in first stage of labor. May be given in second stage if cesarean birth is required.	Assess woman's knowledge regarding the block. Act as advocate to help her obtain further information if needed. Monitor maternal blood pressure to detect the major side effect, which is hypotension. Provide support and comfort.
Spinal-epidural	Vagina, perineum, and uterus	Given in first stage of labor. May be given in second stage if cesarean birth required.	Assess woman's knowledge regarding the block. Act as advocate to help her obtain further information. Monitor maternal vital signs, fetal heart rate, and uterine contractions. Provide support and comfort.
Pudendal	Perineum and lower vagina	Given in second stage just before birth to provide anesthesia for episiotomy or for low forceps delivery.	Assess woman's knowledge regarding the block. Act as advocate to help her obtain further information if needed.
Local infiltration	Perineum	Administered just before birth to provide anesthesia for episiotomy or after birth if a laceration or other repair is needed.	Assess woman's knowledge regarding the block. Provide information as needed. Provide comfort and support. Observe perineum for bruising or other discoloration in the recovery period.

2. Assemble equipment needed to administer the epidural.
3. Begin intravenous (IV) infusion with an 18-gauge plastic indwelling catheter if IV fluids are not already infusing.
4. A bolus of 500–1,000 mL is given before the administration of the epidural to decrease the risk of hypotension.
5. Assist woman to the bathroom to void, provide a bedpan, perform an in and out catheterization, or insert Foley catheter.
6. Assist woman into a side-lying position at edge of bed or in a sitting position with legs over side of bed.
7. The labor nurse or partner supports the woman in this position to help ensure that she does not move during the procedure.
8. The anesthesiologist or certified nurse anesthetist administers the epidural.
9. An indwelling catheter is placed and taped to the woman's back.
10. After the epidural is administered and indwelling catheter is taped, the woman is positioned on her side or in a tilted position to reduce risk of compression of the ascending vena cava and the descending aorta.
- Following the epidural
  1. Assess the woman's ability to lift her legs and the level of sensation every 30 minutes to monitor effects of the nerve block.
  2. The anesthesia level is too high if the woman reports numbness in her chest, face, or tongue or any breathing difficulties.
  3. Assess for bladder distention if Foley catheter was not inserted.
  4. Monitor FHR, contraction pattern, cervical changes, blood pressure, respirations, and temperature per agency protocol.

- If hypotension occurs
  1. Increase IV fluid.
  2. Administer oxygen to increase oxygen concentration to the fetus.
  3. Notify the anesthesiologist or certified nurse anesthetist.
  4. If blood pressure is not restored within 1–2 minutes, administer ephedrine 5–10 mg IV, per physician orders.
- If respiratory rate decreases below 14 respirations per minute, naloxone may be given per physician orders to counteract the effects of the anesthetic agent. See Drug Guide: Naloxone Hydrochloride (Narcan), pp. 301–302.

NURSING CARE AT THE TIME OF BIRTH

- During the second stage of labor the nurse assesses:
  1. Uterine contractions
  2. Fetal status
  3. Maternal blood pressure, pulse, and respirations
  4. Maternal comfort level and need for support during the pushing phase
  5. Needs of support team

See Table 3–5 for nursing assessments during labor and birth.

- Continue encouragement and support of the woman or family.
- Prepare the birthing area when the time of birth approaches.
- Summon the CNM or physician if not already present.
- Continue maternal-fetal assessments as outlined in Table 3–5.
- With support person, assist the woman in her pushing efforts by supporting her legs or shoulders.
- Suggest alternative positions to increase maternal comfort and aid in fetal descent.
- Prepare an instrument table and other equipment.

- Ready oxygen and suction equipment for both mother and newborn if needed.
- Prepare identification bracelets.
- Just before the birth, don sterile gloves and cleanse the perineum.
- Prepare the birth (delivery) bed per CNM/physician preference.

NURSING CARE IMMEDIATELY AFTER THE BIRTH OF THE BABY

During the third stage of labor the nurse assesses both the mother and the newborn.

Apgar Score
- The Apgar score for the newborn is done at 1 and 5 minutes of age.
- Table 3–8 summarizes the Apgar scoring system.

Physical Assessment of the Newborn
- Initial assessment of the newborn includes the following:
    1. Respirations
    2. Apical pulse
    3. Temperature
    4. Skin color
    5. Umbilical cord
    6. Gestational age
    7. Sole creases
    8. Gross fetal abnormalities
- See Table 3–9 for initial newborn evaluation.

Maternal Assessment after Birth
- Assess blood pressure and pulse rate.
- Monitor for signs of placental separation:
    1. Uterus becomes globular in shape and firm.
    2. Uterus rises upward in the abdomen.

Table 3–8 The Apgar Scoring System

Sign	Score 0	Score 1	Score 2
Heart rate	Absent	Slow—below 100	Above 100
Respiratory effort	Absent	Slow, irregular	Good crying
Muscle tone	Flaccid	Some flexion of extremities	Active motion
Reflex irritability	None	Grimace	Vigorous cry
Color	Pale blue	Body pink, blue extremities	Completely pink

Source: From "The Newborn (Apgar) Scoring System: Reflections and Advice," by V. Apgar, August 1966, *Pediatric Clinics of North America, 13*, 645.

   3. Umbilical cord lengthens.

   4. A sudden gush of blood.

- Don disposable gloves when handling the newborn.
- Provide warmth for the newborn by drying with warmed, soft blankets, by placing the newborn under a radiant warmer, or by placing the newborn skin to skin with the mother and removing wet blankets.
- Maintain a clear airway in the newborn by suctioning with the bulb syringe or by using nasopharyngeal suctioning if needed.
- Prevent infection in the newborn by washing hands thoroughly before the birth, maintaining asepsis in placing the umbilical cord clamp, and maintaining asepsis if eye prophylaxis is administered in the birthing area.
- Ensure correct identification of the newborn by placing identification bracelets on the mother and newborn at birth (in some institutions, an identification band is also placed on the support person) and obtaining newborn's footprints and maternal fingerprint on birth record (done in some facilities). A security alarm may also be placed at the same time.
- Continue to provide support to the woman and her partner.
- Maintain birth record for the client chart.

Table 3–9   Initial Newborn Evaluation

Assess	Normal Findings
Respirations	Rate 30–60 irregular No retractions, no grunting
Apical pulse	Rate 110–160 and somewhat irregular
Temperature	Skin temp above 97.8°F (36.5°C)
Skin color	Body pink with bluish extremities
Umbilical cord	Two arteries and one vein
Gestational age	Should be 38–42 weeks to remain with parents for extended time
Sole creases	Sole creases that involve the heel
General assessment	No gross abnormalities

In general, expect scant amount of vernix on upper back, axilla, groin; lanugo only on upper back; ears with incurving of upper two-thirds of pinnae and thin cartilage that springs back from folding; male genitalia—testes palpated in upper or lower scrotum; female genitalia—labia majora larger; clitoris nearly covered.

In the following situations, newborns should generally be stabilized rather than remaining with parents in the birth area for an extended period of time:

- Apgar is less than 8 at 1 minute and less than 9 at 5 minutes, or a baby requires resuscitation measures (other than whiffs of oxygen).
- Respirations are below 30 or above 60, with retractions and/or grunting.
- Apical pulse is below 110 or above 160 with marked irregularities.
- Skin temperature is below 97.8°F (36.5°C).
- Skin color is pale blue, or there is circumoral pallor.
- Baby is less than 38 or more than 42 weeks' gestation.
- Baby is very small or vary large for gestational age.
- There are congenital anomalies involving open areas in the skin (meningomyelocele).

- Monitor maternal blood pressure, pulse, and signs of placental separation.
- Administer oxytocin as ordered by physician or CNM. The oxytocin may be added to the IV solution if one has already been started, or it may be given intramuscularly (frequently the ventrogluteal or vastus lateralis site is used).

NURSING CARE IN THE IMMEDIATE RECOVERY PERIOD

Maternal Assessments in the Fourth Stage

- Assessments are done q15min × 4, q30min × 2, q1–2h × 2.
  1. Assess blood pressure and pulse.
  2. Assess the uterine fundus (Figure 3–5). See Procedures: Assessing the Status of the Uterine Fundus after Birth, pp. 318–321.
  3. After removing the peripad or Chux, observe the perineum for swelling, bruising, or lacerations.
  4. Assess the amount of lochia. See Procedures: Evaluating Lochia, pp. 327–330.
  5. Assess for bladder distention.
- The nurse can anticipate the findings indicated in Table 3–10.

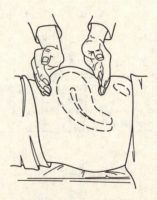

Figure 3–5 ■ Suggested method of palpating the fundus of the uterus during the fourth stage. The left hand is placed just above the symphysis pubis, and gentle downward pressure is exerted. The right hand is cupped around the uterine fundus.

Table 3–10   Maternal Adaptations following Birth

Characteristic	Normal Findings
Blood pressure	Should return to prelabor level
Pulse	Slightly lower than in labor
Uterine fundus	In the midline at the umbilicus or 1–2 finger breadths below the umbilicus
Lochia	Red (rubra), small to moderate amount (from spotting on pads to $1/4$–$1/2$ of pad covered in 15 minutes); should not exceed saturation of one pad in first hour
Bladder	Nonpalpable
Perineum	Smooth, pink, without bruising or edema
Emotional state	Wide variation, including excited, exhilarated, smiling, crying, fatigued, verbal, quiet, pensive, and sleepy

- The frequent assessments of the immediate recovery cease when
  1. Blood pressure and pulse are stable.
  2. Uterus is firm, in the midline, and below the umbilicus.
  3. Lochia is rubra, moderate in amount, without clots.
  4. Perineum is free from bruising or excessive edema.

Maternal Interventions in the Fourth Stage

- Massage uterus if it becomes soft (boggy).
- Assist mother to the bathroom to void.
- Provide warm blankets if mother experiences postpartum chills.
- Provide fluids and food per physician's/CNM's order.
- Encourage the mother and partner to hold the infant as they desire.
- Facilitate eye contact with newborn by turning down the lights in the recovery area.
- Explain newborn characteristics.

Newborn Assessments

- Assessments are done q30min × 2, q1h, and then q8h if stable.
    1. Assess temperature, pulse, and respirations.
    2. Assess skin color.
    3. Observe for signs of cold stress or hypoglycemia.
    4. If large for gestational age (LGA) or small for gestational age (SGA) or infant of a diabetic mother, assess newborn glucose level via heel stick for capillary blood.

Newborn Interventions

- Maintain newborn temperature by placing a warm blanket over newborn, by placing newborn in skin-to-skin contact with mother, or by placing newborn in a radiant-heated unit.
- If newborn is in a radiant-heated unit, he or she is dried, placed on a warm blanket, and left uncovered.
- Suction nose and mouth with a bulb syringe as needed.
- Apply tetracycline or erythromycin ophthalmic ointment in each eye. See Drug Guide: Erythromycin Ophthalmic Ointment, pp. 292–293.
- Give vitamin K_1 mg per physician orders. See Drug Guide: Vitamin K_1 Phytonadione (AquaMephyton), pp. 310–311.
- Initiate breast-feeding if desired by mother.

REFERENCE

Pan American Health Organization. (2006). *Domestic violence during pregnancy*. Retrieved September 26, 2006, from http://www.paho.org.

4 THE AT-RISK INTRAPARTAL CLIENT

FAILURE TO PROGRESS IN LABOR

- Defined as no progress in cervical dilatation or descent of the presenting part during active labor for at least 2 hours
- May be associated with malpresentation (breech, transverse, face, or brow), malposition (occiput posterior), or cephalopelvic disproportion (CPD)
- May also be related to dysfunctional uterine contractions
- Maternal risks
  1. Infection secondary to increased number of vaginal examinations to determine status
  2. Dehydration secondary to inadequate fluid intake
  3. Exhaustion associated with lengthening of the labor
- Fetal risks
  1. Nonreassuring fetal status secondary to maternal dehydration and subsequent hypotension
  2. Infection secondary to maternal infection

Management of Failure to Progress

- Intravenous (IV) fluids may be ordered to rehydrate the laboring woman.
- Clinical evaluation is done to rule out CPD. Physician/ certified nurse-midwife (CNM) evaluates cervical dilatation, fetal descent (station), and fetal position.
  1. An oxytocin infusion may be started.
  2. After 2 hours of adequate uterine contractions, cervical dilatation and fetal station are reevaluated.

If progress has been made, labor continues. If no progress has occurred, cesarean birth is indicated.

- If CPD is ruled out and uterine contractions are less than normal in frequency, duration, and quality (intensity), an oxytocin infusion is started to augment the labor pattern. Placement of an intrauterine pressure catheter can document the intensity of uterine contractions.

Nursing Assessments for Failure to Progress

- Assess fetal vertex for engagement into the maternal pelvis.
- Assess uterine contractions for frequency, duration, and intensity.
- If intensity is less than expected (for this point in labor), and the amount of pain the woman experiences seems out of proportion (feels pain before contraction begins, intense discomfort during contraction, and pain after the contraction is gone), consider the possibility of occiput posterior position.
- Assess cervical dilatation and effacement.
  1. Cervical dilatation usually progresses at 1.5 cm/hour for multiparas and 1.2 cm/hour for primigravidas.
  2. If the cervix becomes edematous and thicker during labor, CPD may be present.
- Assess fetal heart rate (FHR).
- Assess fetal position, presentation, and descent.
- An intrapartal vaginal examination may identify problems such as breech, transverse brow or face presentation, or occiput posterior position.
- Assess for presence of caput (edema of subcutaneous tissues in the top of the fetal head). An enlarging caput may confuse the examiner because it feels like further descent of the fetal head.
- Assess descent of the fetal head by determining station.
- Assess laboring woman for hydration status.
- Assess woman's comfort and coping level.
- Assess support person's level of anxiety, because prolonged labor can be stressful to the support person.

Nursing Diagnoses

- Acute pain related to inability to relax secondary to labor pattern
- Risk for ineffective individual coping related to ineffectiveness of breathing techniques to relieve discomfort

Nursing Interventions for Failure to Progress

- Monitor labor status and fetal status through continuous electronic monitoring of mother and fetus.
- Compare assessment findings to expected norms.
- Assist woman with relaxation and breathing techniques.
- Provide comfort measures such as cool washcloth to face or back massage.
- Monitor oxytocin infusion if ordered by CNM/physician (see Induction of Labor later in this chapter).
- Try alternative maternal positions or activity that might facilitate rotation of fetal head or assist with fetal descent. These include standing or walking, turning to one side, sitting on toilet, hands and knees position, squatting, and taking a warm shower.
- Assist woman to bathroom to void because a full bladder can impede fetal descent.
- Keep the woman and her support team informed of assessment findings and progress.
- Prepare for cesarean birth if indicated.
- Chart assessment findings and nursing and medical interventions.

Sample Nurse's Charting

Contractions every 2½ minutes, 60 sec duration and of strong intensity. Cervical dilatation has remained at 7 cm for 1 hour. FHR BL 140–148 with two accelerations of 15 bpm for 15 sec with fetal movement in the last 20 minutes. Good variability. No decelerations present. Voided 200 mL clear amber urine without difficulty. Taking ice chips at will. Skin turgor and mucus membranes indicate adequate hydration. Breathing with contractions but beginning to cry out at the acme. Dozes between contractions but quickly rouses. Asking "Why is it taking so long? Why am I not making progress?" Partner and family asking to speak with physician regarding treatment plan. Call placed to physician and physician to be here in 5 minutes to see client. P. Gomez, RNC

Evaluation

1. The woman experiences a more effective labor pattern.
2. The woman has increased comfort and decreased anxiety.

PRECIPITOUS BIRTH

- Defined as extremely rapid labor that lasts less than 3 hours from start to finish
- Maternal risks
  1. Lacerations of the cervix, vagina, and/or perineum
  2. Uterine rupture
  3. Amniotic fluid embolism
  4. Postpartal hemorrhage
- Fetal/neonatal risks
  1. Fetal hypoxia
  2. Cerebral trauma

Management of Precipitous Birth

- Continue close medical monitoring.
- Obtain previous obstetric history to identify rapid labor.
- Discontinue oxytocin infusion if woman's labor is being induced or augmented.

Nursing Assessments for Precipitous Birth

- Assess previous labor history if the woman is a multipara.
- Assess contraction status. Be alert for contractions that are more frequent than every 2 minutes and dilatation that progresses faster than normal (more than 1.5 cm/hour).
- Assess fetal status.
- Assess mother's comfort level.
- Assess mother's coping abilities.

Nursing Diagnoses

- Acute pain related to accelerated labor pattern
- Risk for ineffective individual coping related to ineffectiveness of breathing techniques to relieve discomfort

Nursing Interventions
for Precipitous Birth

- Continue electronic monitoring.
- Notify physician or CNM of rapid cervical changes.
- Remain in room to provide support and comfort measures for the woman.
- Instruct woman not to bear down until she is instructed to do so.
- Prepare room for birth. Do not take the foot off the bed or "break" the bed.
- Assist with the birth of the baby if the physician or CNM is not present.
    1. Instruct woman to pant with contractions if fetal head is crowning.
    2. Apply gentle pressure anteriorly against the fetal head to maintain flexion and prevent it from being born too quickly.
    3. Support the perineum by making a U-shape with the other hand and supporting the descending head between contractions to prevent excess tearing and perineal lacerations.
    4. Suction the fetal nares and mouth with a bulb syringe.
    5. Insert two fingers along the back of the fetal neck to check for a nuchal cord. If present, bend the fingers like a fish hook, grasp the cord, and pull it over the baby's head. Most tight cords can be reduced; however, if the cord cannot be slipped over the head, place two clamps on it and cut between the clamps. Unwind the cord from around the neck.
    6. While requesting the woman to push gently, exert gentle downward pressure on the head to assist in

the birth of the anterior shoulder by gently pulling downward. Keep hands over the fetal ears to avoid pulling on the fetal neck. Then, exert gentle upward pressure to assist with the posterior shoulder. Support the rest of the baby's body as it is born.

7. Place newborn on maternal abdomen and dry the baby with soft warm blankets, removing blankets as they become wet.

- Check firmness of the uterus. Observe for excessive maternal bleeding. Leave the placenta in place for CNM/physician delivery.

Complete client records.

Evaluation
- The woman and her baby are closely monitored during labor and a safe birth occurs.
- The woman states that she feels support and enhanced comfort during labor and birth.

GESTATIONAL-AGE-RELATED PROBLEMS
- See Table 4–1.

LABOR COMPLICATED BY MALPRESENTATION OR MALPOSITION
- See Table 4–2.
- See Figure 4–1 for selected types of fetal malpresentations.

PROLAPSED UMBILICAL CORD
- Occurs when the umbilical cord precedes the fetus down the birth canal
- Conditions associated with prolapsed cord
  1. Breech presentation
  2. Transverse lie
  3. Contracted pelvic inlet
  4. Small fetus
  5. Extra long cord

Table 4–1 Babies with Special Needs in Labor and Birth

Type	Implication for Labor	Treatment	Immediate Nursing Support
Postterm	More likely to have decreased amount of amniotic fluid, so variable decelerations are more likely. Meconium may be present in amniotic fluid.	Induction if BPP score decreases, if amniotic fluid volume decreases, or if pregnancy reaches 42 weeks. Amnioinfusion for severe variable decelerations.	Continuous EFM during labor. At birth, assist physician or CNM with visualization of cord and nasopharyngeal suctioning if fluid is meconium stained.
Preterm	Stress of labor is difficult for baby. Parents are very concerned about baby. Analgesia may be withheld to avoid depressing the fetus/newborn.	Tocolytic therapy to suppress labor. Epidural may be given for laboring women.	Have pediatrician, neonatologist, and nursing support available. Provide respiratory support, temperature stabilization, and rapid assessment of newborn.
Multiple gestation	Vertex-vertex presentation is most common, followed by vertex-breech. Increased risk of prolapsed cord and cord entanglement.	Vaginal birth of vertex-vertex presentation may be possible. Other presentations may be possible with guided ultrasound. Continuous EFM of both babies during labor.	For vaginal birth or cesarean birth, double numbers of personnel are required. Provide respiratory support and temperature stabilization.
Macrosomia (weight greater than 4,000 g)	CPD is more likely. Dysfunctional labor due to overstretching of uterine muscle fibers. Shoulder dystocia most serious complication.	If CPD present, then cesarean birth performed. If shoulder dystocia suspected, position woman in McRoberts' position.	Baby is more likely to develop hypoglycemia. If shoulder dystocia, assess for shoulder movement and crepitus over clavicle.

BPP, biophysical profiles; CNM, certified nurse-midwife; CPD, cephalopelvic disproportion; EFM, electronic fetal monitor.

Table 4–2   Impact of Fetal Malpresentation or Malposition on Birth

Fetal Position	Implication for Labor	Treatment Needed or Anticipated	Nursing Interventions	Impact on Newborn
Occiput posterior	Labor may be longer. Severe back pain may be present.	Forceps, manual rotation, or vacuum at birth may be needed.	Apply sacral pressure. Apply hot packs to sacral area. Monitor labor maternal-fetal status. Assist mother into hands-and-knees position and instruct her to do pelvic rock. Alternative position would be to put weight on knees and lean over raised head of bed, change position from side to side, squat, and/or sit on a toilet.	If labor is longer, fetus is more likely to experience nonreassuring fetal status. Head is molded.
Brow presentation (see Figure 4–1)	Labor may be longer.	If CPD is suspected or present, and labor is arrested, then cesarean birth is appropriate.	Monitor labor maternal-fetal status. Provide support measures. Assist with cesarean birth if indicated.	—

Face presentation (see Figure 4–1)	Risks of CPD and prolonged labor are increased.	If no CPD is present and chin (mentum) is anterior, vaginal birth may be possible. If chin is posterior, a cesarean birth is necessary.	Monitor labor and maternal-fetal status. Provide support measures. Assist with cesarean birth if indicated.	—
Breech (see Figure 4–1)	Labor may be prolonged. Meconium may be expelled in amniotic fluid.	External version may be done at 36–38 weeks and then vaginal birth. If version unsuccessful, cesarean birth is scheduled. Some obstetricians may consider vaginal birth for frank breech.	Monitor labor and maternal-fetal status. Monitor for prolapsed cord.	May develop facial edema during labor. May have edema of throat that compromises breathing. Newborn has increased risk of mortality and intracranial hemorrhage from traumatic birth of head during vaginal birth. Brachial plexus palsy may occur with vaginal birth.

CPD, cephalopelvic disproportion.

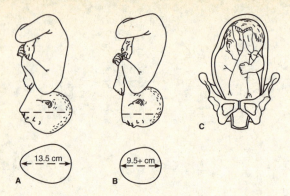

Figure 4–1 ■ Types of malpresentation. **A,** Brow presentation: the largest anterior-posterior diameter presents to the maternal pelvis. **B,** Face presentation: vaginal birth may be possible if the fetal chin is toward the maternal symphysis pubis. **C,** Breech presentation.

6. Low-lying placenta
7. Hydramnios
8. Twin gestations
9. Nonengaged presenting part
- Fetal/neonatal risks
  1. Decreased oxygenation and circulation related to the compressed umbilical cord, with possible non-reassuring fetal status

Management of Prolapsed Cord

- Recognize early.
- Once prolapsed cord is identified, an emergency cesarean birth is usually indicated.

Nursing Assessments for Prolapsed Cord

- Assess woman's present pregnancy for conditions associated with prolapsed cord.
- Assess FHR via electronic fetal monitor (EFM), because cord compression is associated with variable

decelerations and periodic auscultation may or may not identify a variable deceleration.

- Assess for presence of cord prolapse via intrapartal vaginal exam.
- *Be alert for* the presence of a pulsating, slick cord (see Figure 4–2).

Nursing Diagnoses

- Risk for alteration in gas exchange in the fetus related to decreased blood flow secondary to compression of the umbilical cord
- Fear related to unknown outcome

Nursing Interventions for Prolapsed Cord

- Complete an intrapartal vaginal examination to check for prolapse of the cord when variable decelerations are noted on EFM tracing and/or after membranes have ruptured. (See Procedure: Performing an Intrapartal Vaginal Examination, pp. 338–342.)
- Relieve pressure of the fetal presenting part by leaving the gloved fingers in the vagina and lifting the fetal head off the cord (push fetus up toward the body of the uterus).

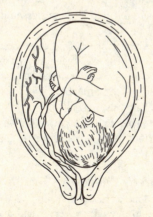

Figure 4–2 ■ Prolapse of the umbilical cord.

- Call for assistance. Other nurses can assist in the preparation of the woman for emergency cesarean birth. The CNM/physician should be STAT paged.
- If possible, place woman in knee-chest or Trendelenburg position.
- Maintain the maternal position and pressure on the fetal presenting part until the CNM/physician arrives and/or a cesarean birth is accomplished.
- In some instances, an indwelling bladder catheter may be inserted to fill the bladder with warmed normal saline. The filled bladder places upward pressure on the fetal presenting part and relieves pressure on the cord.
- Administer oxygen to the mother by face mask at 7–10 L/minute.
- Provide information and support to the laboring couple.
- Review the following critical aspects of the care you have provided:
  1. What is the response of the FHR to the intervention?
  2. Has the rate returned to the range of 110–160 beats per minute?
  3. Is there evidence of variable decelerations on the EFM tracing?
  4. Are the variable decelerations lessening in depth or number?
  5. Is the position I have asked the woman to assume working? Is FHR improving? Can this position be maintained until a cesarean birth can be accomplished?
  6. Is the baby moving much?
  7. Are accelerations present?
  8. What do I need to protect myself from the woman's bodily fluids? Can a colleague tie a plastic apron around me?

Sample Nurse's Charting

Vaginal exam done to assess dilatation status. Prolapse of the umbilical cord through the cervix and into the vagina. Immediate pressure placed on the fetal vertex. EFM monitor indicates FHR maintained BL of 144–150 from beginning of exam throughout intervention. Variability average. Accelerations of 20 bpm for 15 sec with fetal movement and palpation of fetus. Immediate call placed to Dr. to advise of status. IV of 1,000 mL lactated Ringer's started in R wrist after one attempt with 18 ga Quik cath. Running at 125 mL/hr. 16Fr indwelling Foley catheter inserted. Abdominal-perineal prep done. To surgery for emergency cesarean birth. Continuous pressure placed on fetal vertex through the vagina until birth. Permit signed by husband. P. Gomez, RNC

HYDRAMNIOS

- Occurs when there is over 2,000 mL of amniotic fluid in the amniotic sac.
- Exact cause is unknown; however, hydramnios can occur in cases of major congenital anomalies, maternal diabetes, infections, and alloimmunization.
- Maternal risks
  1. Shortness of breath
  2. Edema in the lower extremities from compression of the vena cava
- Fetal/neonatal risks
  1. Increased risk of mortality due to an increased prevalence of fetal malformations associated with hydramnios
  2. Increased incidence of preterm birth
  3. Increased incidence of malpresentation
  4. Increased incidence of prolapse of the cord

Management of Hydramnios

- Provide supportive therapy.
- Assess fundal size and monitor growth throughout pregnancy.
- Complete ultrasound examinations to determine presence of anomalies and measure amniotic fluid volume.
- Decrease amount of amniotic fluid. In some instances, an amniocentesis may be done to remove fluid in order to reduce the risk of preterm labor.

Nursing Assessments for Hydramnios

- Assess woman's history for other associated problems, such as diabetes, Rh sensitization, fetal malformations, infections during the intrapartum period, or multiple gestation.
- Assess FHR. It may be more difficult to auscultate the FHR because of the increased amount of fluid. Placement of the EFM may also be more difficult because of the size of the maternal abdomen.
- Be alert for the presence of variable decelerations that may indicate prolapse of the cord.
- Assess maternal blood pressure (BP) for hypotension related to compression of the vena cava.
- Assess respiratory rate because weight of the uterus can compromise maternal circulation.
- Assess for fetal malpresentation-malposition by intrapartal vaginal examination of the presenting part.

Nursing Diagnoses

- Risk for impaired gas exchange related to pressure on the diaphragm secondary to hydramnios
- Fear related to unknown outcome of the pregnancy

Nursing Interventions for Hydramnios

- Position woman on her left or right side.
- Monitor maternal and fetal status frequently. (See Table 3–5, p. 91.)
- Because of increased incidence of fetal problems, continuous EFM may be warranted.
- Monitor amount of amniotic fluid lost and characteristics of fluid.
- Be alert for presence of meconium in the fluid, which may be associated with nonreassuring fetal status.

Evaluation

- Maternal and fetal status remains stable, with BP, pulse, respirations, and FHR in normal ranges.
- Woman reports that her questions have been answered and her fears have been addressed.

OLIGOHYDRAMNIOS

- Occurs when the amount of amniotic fluid is severely reduced and concentrated.
- Exact cause is unknown; however, oligohydramnios is found in cases of postmaturity, with intrauterine growth restriction (IUGR) secondary to placental insufficiency, and in fetal conditions associated with renal and urinary malfunction.
- Maternal risks
  1. Dysfunctional labor
- Fetal risks
  1. Fetal hypoxia associated with compression of the umbilical cord because the umbilical cord has less fluid surrounding it
  2. Increased risk of pulmonary hypoplasia if oligohydramnios has been present throughout the gestation

Management of Oligohydramnios

- Oligohydramnios is usually identified by serial ultrasound examinations during pregnancy.
- Amnioinfusion (infusion of warmed saline solution) may be done during labor after the membranes have ruptured to decrease the risk of cord compression.
- Monitor fetus with daily fetal movement counts, nonstress testing (NST), and biophysical profiles.
- Monitor fetal status.
- Increase maternal hydration and maintain bedrest.

Nursing Assessments
for Oligohydramnios

- Assess the results of any prenatal testing that indicates decreased amniotic fluid volume:
  1. Ultrasound exam with notations of decreased volume
  2. Biophysical profile (BPP) score that is decreased because of diminished amniotic fluid volume
  3. Nonreactive NSTs due to fetal decelerations because of cord compression

- Assess FHR.
  1. *Be alert for* variable decelerations.
  2. If membranes rupture, note color and amount of fluid.
- Assess for the presence of meconium.

Nursing Diagnoses
- Risk for impaired gas exchange related to pressure on the umbilical cord secondary to decreased amniotic fluid
- Fear related to unknown outcome of pregnancy

Nursing Interventions for Oligohydramnios
- Monitor maternal status on a frequent basis:
  1. Watch for hypotension.
  2. Assess for anxiety and tension.
- Monitor fetal status on a frequent basis for signs of decreased placental-fetal profusion. *Be alert for* presence of variable decelerations and decreased variability.
- Encourage woman to maintain side-lying position while in bed.
- Assist with amnioinfusion if done.

Evaluation
- The woman and her partner state that they understand the condition, the need for monitoring, and possible associated problems.
- The woman gives birth to a healthy newborn.

AMNIOTIC FLUID EMBOLISM
- Catastrophic event that occurs when a small amount of amniotic fluid enters the maternal bloodstream. The amniotic fluid moves through the maternal circulation, through the right atrium and ventricle, and then into the pulmonary circulation.
- Maternal mortality rate is approximately 70% (Cunningham et al., 2005).
- Symptoms may include the following:
  1. Sudden respiratory distress
  2. Tachycardia
  3. Circulatory collapse

4. Acute hemorrhage
5. Cor pulmonale
6. Hypotension
7. Shock
8. Coma

- Fetal hypoxia or anoxia occurs as the mother experiences respiratory difficulty or respiratory arrest.

Management of Amniotic Fluid Embolism

- Emergency support measures, which may include intubation, are instituted.
- Immediate intensive care to support circulatory and respiratory systems is required.
- Oxygen is administered by mask or positive pressure.
- Intravenous (IV) therapy is begun.
- Central hemodynamic monitoring lines are necessary to monitor pressures and make treatment decisions.
- Dopamine may be required to maintain maternal BP.
- Coagulation studies are completed to monitor the development of disseminated intravascular coagulation (DIC) and to monitor treatment.
- Continuous EFM is necessary to monitor fetal status.
- Immediate birth via cesarean section may be warranted.

Nursing Assessments for Amniotic Fluid Embolism

- Assess for associated factors such as multiparity, hydramnios, tumultuous labor (contractions with frequency of less than 2 minutes and strong intensity). Tumultuous labor may occur naturally or may be associated with IV oxytocin administration.
- Assess maternal vital signs.
- *Be alert for* signs of respiratory distress or any statement from the mother that she is experiencing difficulty breathing.
- Assess FHR for rate, variability, and presence of decelerations.
- Assess for hemorrhage and signs of shock.

Nursing Diagnoses

- Risk for impaired gas exchange related to cardiopulmonary collapse
- Fear related to risk of death secondary to pulmonary embolism

Nursing Interventions for Amniotic Fluid Embolism

- Continuously monitor and evaluate maternal-fetal status.
- If respiratory difficulties occur:
  1. Provide oxygen.
  2. Call for emergency assistance. Provide respiratory and cardiac support until assistance arrives.
  3. Start one or two peripheral IV lines.
  4. Prepare for administration of whole blood.
  5. Prepare for insertion of central venous pressure (CVP) line.
  6. Monitor fluid intake.
  7. Assist with emergency measures.
  8. Have one nurse note the type and administration time of all medications.
- Complete client records. Nurses' notes need to reflect the time symptoms began, what the signs and symptoms were, the actions taken, and the response of the client. Continuing assessments are also documented.
- Prepare for emergency cesarean birth.

Evaluation

- The mother and baby are monitored carefully.
- Emergency measures are instituted immediately.

ABRUPTIO PLACENTAE IN THE INTRAPARTAL PERIOD

- Defined as premature separation of the placenta from the uterine wall.
- Signs and symptoms: see Table 4–3 for characteristics of placenta previa and abruptio placentae.

Table 4–3   Characteristics of Placenta Previa and Abruptio Placentae

Placenta Previa	Abruptio Placentae
Bright red bleeding	May be bright red or dark red in color, or no bleeding may be apparent if abruption is concealed.
No pain	May have no pain if abruption was on margin of placenta and has now resolved.
May have history of painless, bright red bleeding	May have pain if abruption is central (behind placenta). If contractions are present, may have increased tonus of uterus and poor uterine relaxation between contractions. Uterus may be "board-like."

- Maternal risks
  1. Maternal mortality rate is approximately 6%
  2. Hemorrhage and development of DIC
  3. Renal failure due to shock
  4. Vascular spasm
- Fetal/neonatal risks
  1. Preterm labor
  2. Anemia
  3. Hypoxia

Management of Abruptio Placentae

- Mild abruption (vaginal bleeding absent or external bleeding of less than 100 mL): The labor can continue and vaginal birth is anticipated.
- Moderate abruption (vaginal bleeding absent or from 100–500 mL) and severe abruption (vaginal bleeding absent or greater than 500 mL):
  1. Continuous monitoring of the mother and fetus
  2. Monitoring and treatment of shock
  3. Evaluation of coagulation
  4. Possible blood replacement
  5. If indicated, amniotomy and oxytocin infusion to induce or augment labor

- Cesarean birth is indicated when:
  1. Nonreassuring fetal status develops and a vaginal birth is not imminent.
  2. The fetus is alive and a severe abruption occurs.
  3. Hemorrhage becomes severe and threatens the life of the mother.
  4. Labor is not progressing.

Nursing Assessments for Abruptio Placentae

- Assess maternal history for associated factors:
  1. Preeclampsia or chronic hypertension
  2. High multiparity
  3. Trauma/domestic violence
  4. Use of illicit drugs such as cocaine or crack
- Assess type and amount of bleeding to assist in differentiating among possible causes of bleeding.
- Pads may be weighed to assess blood loss more accurately (1 g equals 1 mL). Hemorrhage of 500 mL or more increases chance of fetal death.
- Assess whether pain is present:
  1. Pain is present in most women with abruptio placentae.
  2. The pain is usually of sudden onset, is constant, and is localized to the uterus or the lower back.
  3. Determine if the pain is associated with uterine contractions. Is there pain between contractions (feels as if the uterus stays tight and does not relax)?
  4. Determine if there are tender areas over the uterus.
- Assess uterine contractions for frequency, duration, intensity, and resting tone between contractions. (Abruptio placentae is associated with a rising uterine tone baseline.)
- Assess size of uterus. If bleeding is concealed, the uterus may be filling with blood and the fundus will rise.
- Assess labor progress for cervical dilatation, effacement, and fetal station. (Abruption may be associated with precipitous birth.)

- Assess maternal vital signs.
- Assess fetal status by EFM.
- Assess laboratory studies (hemoglobin, hematocrit, DIC screen).

Nursing Diagnoses
- Fluid volume deficit related to hypovolemia secondary to excessive blood loss
- Anxiety related to concern for personal health and the baby's safety

Nursing Interventions for Abruptio Placentae
- Monitor maternal status. *Be alert for* beginning signs of shock (decreased BP, increased pulse, increased respirations).
- Monitor fetal status. *Be alert for* FHR baseline changes and late decelerations with decreased variability.
- Monitor amount of blood loss:
  1. Measure blood loss.
  2. Wear disposable gloves when handling blood-soaked items or while cleansing blood from woman.
- Carefully monitor labor status. *Be alert for* increased uterine tonus, which may be exhibited by
  1. Increased frequency of contractions (less than 2 minutes)
  2. Increased intensity
  3. Incomplete uterine relaxation between contractions
  4. Tenderness of the uterine fundus
  5. A rising baseline of EFM strip
- Monitor urine output. Urine output is reflective of circulatory status.
  1. Urine output needs to be at least 30 mL/hour.
  2. An indwelling bladder catheter will assist in monitoring urine output accurately.
  3. Amount of output is measured every 1–4 hours, depending on the severity of the bleeding.

- Monitor size of abdomen:
  1. Place measuring tape under woman; then bring it around to the front and over the umbilicus.
  2. Use either the upper or lower edge of the umbilicus and, for consistency, consider making marks on the maternal abdomen with a felt-tip pen to ensure consistent placement of the tape in each measurement.
- Monitor oxytocin if it is being administered. See Induction of Labor later in this chapter.
- Monitor laboratory studies. *Be alert for* development of consumption coagulopathy (DIC) as evidenced by decreasing platelets and fibrinogen and increased fibrin split products (see Table 4–4).
- Monitor oxygen status by pulse oximetry (pulse oximetry needs to be 95 or above). If reading is below 95, administer oxygen by face mask at 7–10 L/minute.
- Monitor fluid and blood replacement.
- Monitor for signs of decreased platelet count such as purpura, petechiae, bruising, hematemesis, and rectal bleeding.
- Prepare for cesarean birth if vaginal birth is not imminent.
- Follow standard precautions and Centers for Disease Control and Prevention (CDC) precautions at all times of exposure to body fluids.
- Provide emotional support for woman and her support team.

Table 4–4   Laboratory Findings Associated with Disseminated Intravascular Coagulation (DIC)

Lab Test	Normal Value	Value in DIC
Partial thromboplastin	60–70 sec	Prolonged
Platelets	150,000–400,000 mcL	Decreased
Fibrinogen	200–400 mg/dL	Decreased
Fibrin degradation products (also called fibrin split products or fibrin)	2–10 mcg/mL	Increased

- Review the following critical aspects of the care you have provided:
  1. Are the woman's vital signs stable?
  2. Are the vital signs responding in an anticipated way to the medical therapy?
  3. What does the woman say about her condition?
  4. Is she anxious?
  5. Is the amount of bleeding increasing?
  6. What are the measured amounts of blood loss?
  7. Is there bleeding from any other site?
  8. Is the uterus becoming more tender and/or more sensitive?
  9. Is there a rising uterine resting tone?
  10. Is there a better position to place the woman in to maximize circulation and comfort?
  11. What other pieces of information do the woman and her loved ones need?
  12. Has there been a change in her consciousness level?

Sample Nurse's Charting

Uterine contractions every 3 min, 60 sec duration and strong intensity. Uterus relaxes between contractions. Client reports slight tenderness in the upper uterine fundus on the right when palpated. FHR 140–146, decreased variability, no accelerations with fetal movement. Deceleration of 15 bpm lasting 15 sec begins just after acme of each contraction. O_2 per face mask at 8 L/min. Client lying on left side. BP stable at 112/70. Admitting BP 114/72. Pulse 80 and regular. 100 cc dark red vaginal bleeding present on chux in last hour. Client breathing with contractions and relaxing well with encouragement. Partner provides continuous, ongoing support. Dr. Jones here with client. P. Gomez, RNC

Evaluation

- The woman and her baby have a safe labor and birth without further complications.
- The woman and family verbalize understanding of reasons for medical therapy and risks.

PLACENTA PREVIA
IN THE INTRAPARTAL PERIOD

- Implantation of the placenta in the lower uterine segment rather than the upper portion of the uterus
- May occur as:
  1. Low placental implantation
  2. Partial or marginal previa
  3. Complete previa
- Maternal risks
  1. Hemorrhage
  2. Possible complications of emergency cesarean birth
- Fetal/neonatal risks
  1. Anemia due to maternal blood loss
  2. Hypoxia due to maternal blood loss

Management of Placenta Previa

- Diagnosis made from ultrasound examination.
- Cesarean birth scheduled if complete previa, gestation greater than 37 weeks, and documented fetal maturity.
- Labor and vaginal birth may be possible if marginal placenta previa.

Nursing Assessments for Placenta Previa

- Assess type and amount of bleeding (see Table 4–3 for characteristics of placenta previa and abruptio placentae).
- Assess maternal vital signs and fetal status.
- Assess labor progress (uterine contraction frequency, duration, and intensity; fetal descent).
- Assess laboratory findings.

Nursing Diagnoses

- Risk for altered tissue perfusion related to blood loss
- Risk for impaired fetal gas exchange related to decreased blood volume and hypotension
- Anxiety related to concern for own personal status and the baby's safety

Nursing Interventions
for Placenta Previa

- Monitor bleeding. Weigh all absorbent pads to determine amount of blood loss.
- Monitor maternal vital signs for signs of shock.
- Monitor FHR for evidence of normality (baseline stable, variability average, no periodic decelerations or early decelerations).
- Note signs of possible fetal problems such as rising or falling baseline, decreased variability, and late and/or variable decelerations.
- Monitor laboratory studies.
  1. *Be alert for* evidence of decreasing hemoglobin and hematocrit.
  2. Coagulation problems are not as common with placenta previa as with abruptio placentae.
- Administer and monitor IV fluids and blood replacement.
- Monitor oxygen status. If vital signs are unstable or questionable, monitor pulse oximetry. If pulse oximetry is below 95, administer oxygen by face mask at 7–10 L/min.
- Maintain on bed rest with bathroom privileges.
- Provide emotional support to mother and support team.

Evaluation

- Maternal hemorrhage ceases and any hypovolemia is corrected as indicated by normal blood studies and normal maternal vital signs.
- Signs of nonreassuring fetal status are recognized promptly, and corrective measures are begun.

DIABETES MELLITUS (DM) IN THE INTRAPARTUM PERIOD

- Endocrine disorder of carbohydrate metabolism resulting from inadequate production or use of insulin. It may be a preexisting condition or may develop during pregnancy (gestational diabetes mellitus [see Chapter 2]).

- Maternal risks
  1. Increased incidence of preeclampsia
  2. Hypoglycemia
  3. Infection
  4. Diabetic ketoacidosis
  5. Hypertension
  6. Prolonged labor due to CPD
  7. Prolapsed cord related to hydramnios
  8. Hypertonic contractions
  9. Amniotic fluid embolism
  10. Postpartum hemorrhage due to uterine atony
- Fetal/neonatal risks
  1. Fetal macrosomia
  2. Birth trauma related to fetal macrosomia
  3. Increase of congenital abnormalities
  4. Nonreassuring fetal status related to decreased uteroplacental function
  5. Intrauterine fetal demise
  6. Small for gestational age (SGA) if uteroplacental insufficiency present

Intrapartal Management of Diabetes Mellitus

- Induction of labor at 40 weeks if labor does not begin spontaneously
- IV therapy with 5% dextrose in lactated Ringer's solution
- Insulin infusion (rate determined by plasma glucose levels)
- Blood glucose levels every hour
- Continuous EFM
- Assessment for CPD
- Neonatologist present at birth

Intrapartal Nursing Assessments for Diabetes Mellitus

- Review woman's prenatal record for the following:
  1. Fetal gestational age

2. Lecithin-sphingomyelin (L/S) ratio and presence of prostaglandin (PG)
3. Degree of glycemic control
4. Medical or obstetrical complications

- Monitor blood glucose levels hourly or as ordered.
- Assess FHR continuously with EFM.
- Assess labor progress—uterine contractions, cervical changes, and fetal descent.
- Assess for signs of preeclampsia.
- Following childbirth, assess for uterine atony.

Nursing Diagnoses

- Fear related to impact of diabetes on maternal and fetal well-being
- Risk for complications related to hypoglycemia or hyperglycemia
- Altered uteroplacental tissue perfusion related to diabetic vascular changes

Intrapartal Nursing Interventions for Diabetes Mellitus

- Monitor blood glucose via finger sticks.
- Observe for signs of hypoglycemia or hyperglycemia.
- Regulate IV per physician's orders.
- Regulate insulin therapy per physician's orders.
- Maintain woman in side-lying position to increase uteroplacental flow.
- Evaluate labor progress for failure to progress or evidence of CPD.
- Evaluate EFM tracing for late deceleration and/or decreased variability.
- Assess newborn for congenital problems.
- Reassure woman and her support team.

Evaluation

- Woman experiences decreased anxiety related to her health and her baby's health status.

- Woman's blood glucose levels remain within normal ranges.
- FHR is within normal limits, with average variability and no late decelerations.

PREECLAMPSIA-ECLAMPSIA IN THE INTRAPARTUM PERIOD

- Defined as a hypertensive disorder of pregnancy.
- Signs and symptoms
  1. Hypertension
  2. Proteinuria
  3. Edema
  4. Hyperreflexia
  5. Headaches
  6. Visual disturbances
  7. Seizures
- Maternal risks
  1. Cerebral hemorrhage, edema, and thrombosis
  2. Thrombocytopenia
  3. Pulmonary edema
  4. Oliguria and renal failure
  5. Hepatic injury
  6. Seizures and coma
  7. Abruptio placentae
  8. DIC
  9. Maternal death
- Fetal/neonatal risks
  1. IUGR
  2. Nonreassuring fetal status related to placental insufficiency or abruptio placentae
  3. Preterm birth

Intrapartal Management of Preeclampsia-Eclampsia

  1. Begin IV magnesium sulfate therapy.
  2. Evaluate fetal status.

3. Monitor BP and reflexes.
4. Ensure pediatrician or neonatal practitioner is present at birth.

Intrapartal Nursing Assessments for Preeclampsia-Eclampsia

- Assess uterine contraction pattern.
- Assess FHR.
- Assess vital signs.
- Assess deep tendon reflexes (DTRs).
- Assess level of consciousness.
- Assess intake and output.
- Assess degree of edema.
- Assess urinary protein with each voiding.

Nursing Diagnoses

- Risk for injury related to the possibility of seizures secondary to cerebral vasospasm or edema
- Injury to fetus related to uteroplacental insufficiency
- Fluid volume excess related to renal injury

Intrapartal Nursing Interventions for Preeclampsia-Eclampsia

- Start and monitor IV magnesium sulfate therapy by infusion pump. (See Drug Guide: Magnesium Sulfate, pp. 294–297.)
- Piggyback magnesium sulfate line into main line.
- Observe for signs of magnesium toxicity (decreased respirations, diminished or absent reflexes, drooling, difficulty swallowing, marked lethargy).
- Have calcium gluconate at bedside as antidote for magnesium sulfate overdose.
- Maintain intake and output record.
- Chart BP, respirations, and reflexes every hour.
- Obtain magnesium blood levels per physician's orders.
- Alert physician immediately if magnesium levels elevated or less than therapeutic range.

- Maintain a quiet, dark labor room.
- Limit visitors.

Evaluation
- The woman suffers no eclamptic seizures.
- The woman gives birth to a healthy newborn.

INDUCTION OF LABOR
- Defined as the stimulation of uterine contractions before the spontaneous onset of labor
- Indications for induction
  1. Diabetes mellitus
  2. Renal disease
  3. Preeclampsia-eclampsia
  4. Premature rupture of membranes
  5. History of precipitous labor and birth
  6. Chorioamnionitis
  7. Postterm gestation
  8. Mild abruptio placentae with no nonreassuring fetal status
  9. Intrauterine fetal demise (IUFD)
  10. IUGR
  11. Rh alloimmunization
- Contraindications for induction
  1. Client refusal
  2. Placenta previa or vasa previa
  3. Transverse fetal lie
  4. Prior classic uterine incision
  5. Active genital herpes infection
  6. Some instances of positive human immunodeficiency virus (HIV) status
  7. CPD
  8. Nonreassuring fetal status; presence of FHR late decelerations
- Maternal risks
  1. Water intoxication
  2. Rapid labor and birth

3. Cervical, vaginal, and/or perineal lacerations
- Fetal/neonatal risks
    1. Rapid intracranial pressure changes if rapid labor and birth occur
    2. Decreased placental-fetal circulation if labor pattern is overstimulated
- The most frequent methods of induction are amniotomy, IV administration of oxytocin, or both.
- Prostaglandin E_2 is currently being used for labor priming (softening of the cervix) at term but is not used to induce labor at that time. (See Drug Guide: Dinoprostone [Cervidil] Vaginal Insert, pp. 290–292.)
- For oxytocin induction, 1,000 mL of solution (such as lactated Ringer's) is started IV by a large-bore plastic IV catheter (18 or 20 gauge). Ten units of Pitocin are added to a second 1,000-mL bottle of IV fluid (second bottle needs to match the other primary IV). Other combinations may be used in some facilities. The IV containing the Pitocin is the secondary bottle, and this bottle is administered via an infusion pump.

Nursing Assessments during Induction of Labor

- Assess woman's knowledge and understanding regarding the induction procedure, associated nursing care, and the risks and benefits.
- Assess for any contraindications to the induction procedure.
- Assess maternal vital signs to provide a baseline for further assessments.
- Assess FHR characteristics after obtaining a 20-minute EFM strip.
- Assess FHR for reassuring characteristics (baseline 110–160 beats per minute, average variability, accelerations with fetal movement, no late or variable decelerations present).
- Assess maternal vital signs, contraction pattern and characteristics, cervical dilatation, and fetal response

to IV oxytocin once infusion has begun and with each planned increase in the infusion rate.
- Assess maternal physiologic and psychologic response to uterine contractions.

Nursing Diagnoses
- Health-seeking behavior: information about induction related to an expressed desire to understand the procedure and its implications
- Risk for altered placental tissue perfusion related to potential hypertonic contraction pattern

Nursing Interventions during Induction of Labor
- Provide information to meet knowledge needs of woman and her partner.
- Prepare IV solution and obtain equipment for induction.
- Administer oxytocin as a secondary infusion and increase infusion pump rate according to CNM or physician order.
- Monitor contraction and cervical dilatation pattern and EFM tracing.
  1. If contractions occur more frequently than every 2 minutes, decrease the infusion rate.
  2. If nonreassuring fetal status occurs (decreasing variability, decreasing baseline, or presence of late decelerations), discontinue oxytocin infusion and infuse primary IV solution, institute supportive nursing care (assist to side-lying position, monitor for hypotension, and initiate oxygen), and notify CNM or physician of adverse effects.
- Monitor maternal vital signs, contraction pattern, cervical dilatation status, and EFM tracing on a periodic basis and before any increase of oxytocin.
- Provide supportive nursing measures to increase maternal comfort.
- Advocate for the laboring woman when she requests analgesia or anesthesia block.

- Advise CNM or physician of maternal and fetal conditions frequently.
- Carefully evaluate the need for changes in the infusion rate of oxytocin (increase, decrease, or maintain rate) once an active labor pattern is present.

Evaluation
- Woman verbalizes understanding of the medication utilized, the need to take vital signs frequently, and the need for continuing fetal monitoring to evaluate contractions and fetal response.
- Woman experiences contraction pattern that remains within normal limits.

OBSTETRIC PROCEDURE: EXTERNAL VERSION
- Version is done to change the fetal presentation from breech or transverse to cephalic. It is usually scheduled after the 37th week of pregnancy but may be done in the 39th or 40th.

Nursing Assessments during External Version
- Assess the mother for presence of contraindications (nonreactive nonstress test [NST], evidence of CPD, multiple gestation, oligohydramnios, ruptured amniotic membranes, and placenta previa).
- Assess maternal BP, pulse, and respirations.
- Assess FHR (establish presence of reassuring characteristics: FHR baseline between 110 and 160 beats per minute, moderate to average variability, absence of late or variable decelerations).

Nursing Diagnosis
- Health-seeking behavior: information about external version related to an expressed desire to understand the procedure, its risks, and its benefits.

Nursing Interventions during External Version

- Provide information regarding the version.
- Determine woman's Rh status. If she is Rh negative, obstetrician will probably order a minidose of Rh immune globulin (RhoGAM).
- Monitor maternal BP and pulse before the version and every 5 minutes during the procedure.
- Administer tocolytic per physician order.
- Monitor FHR continuously during the version.
- Provide support to the woman and her partner.
- Provide aftercare instructions that may include maternal monitoring for contractions and fetal movement (fetal kick counts).

Evaluation

- The version is accomplished successfully, with no complications.

OBSTETRIC PROCEDURE: FORCEPS-ASSISTED BIRTH

- Indications
  1. Used for rotation of the fetus when there is a persistent posterior position or transverse arrest (anterior-posterior diameters of the fetal head remain transverse in the maternal pelvis)
  2. Used for traction to assist birth
- Contraindications
  1. CPD
  2. Incomplete dilatation of the cervix
  3. Unengaged fetal head
- Maternal risks
  1. Laceration of the cervix, vagina, or perineum
  2. Hematoma
  3. Extension of episiotomy into rectum
  4. Rupture of uterus

- Fetal/neonatal risks
  1. Facial edema and/or bruising
  2. Neurologic injury related to skull fracture or intracranial hemorrhage

Nursing Assessments during Forceps-Assisted Birth
- Assess maternal ability to relax perineal muscles during forceps application and use.
- Assess maternal vital signs.
- Assess contraction pattern.
- Assess fetal status.
- Assess for contraindications.

Nursing Diagnoses
- Health-seeking behavior: lack of understanding of the procedure and its possible complications
- Ineffective individual coping related to unexpected labor progress and use of procedure

Nursing Interventions during Forceps-Assisted Birth
- Explain procedure to mother and partner.
- Monitor woman's comfort and coping level.
- Monitor uterine contractions and inform physician of presence of contractions.
- Monitor FHR after each contraction or continuously by EFM.
- Provide emotional support for the woman and her partner.
- Assess newborn immediately after birth for possible injuries related to forceps-assisted birth.

Evaluation
- Mother and partner understand procedure and possible complications.
- Mother and baby experience no complications.

OBSTETRIC PROCEDURE: VACUUM-ASSISTED BIRTH (VACUUM EXTRACTION)

- Vacuum-assisted birth is an obstetric procedure used to facilitate the birth of a fetus.
- Indications: used for traction to assist birth.
- Contraindications
  1. CPD
  2. Face or breech presentation
- Fetal/neonatal risks
  1. Fetal scalp bruising and/or blistering
  2. Cerebral trauma
- Procedure
  1. The physician places a suction cup on the fetal scalp.
  2. Tubing from the suction cup is attached to the suction device.
  3. The nurse usually initiates suction.
  4. The physician applies traction during contractions.
  5. Suction pressure is decreased between contractions.
- Nursing assessments, diagnoses, interventions, and evaluation are similar to those in forceps-assisted birth.

REFERENCES

Cunningham, F. G., Leveno, K. J., Bloom, S., Hauth, J. C., Gilstrap, L. C., & Wenstrom, K. D. (2005). *Williams obstetrics* (22nd ed.). Stamford, CT: Appleton & Lange.

5 THE NORMAL NEWBORN

At the moment of birth, numerous physiologic adaptations begin to take place in the newborn's body. Because of these dramatic changes, the newborn requires close observation to determine how smoothly she or he is making the transition to extrauterine life. The newborn also requires care that enhances her or his chances of making the transition successfully. The broad goals of nursing care during this period are to provide comprehensive care to the newborn while she or he is in the nursery, to teach parents how to care for their new baby, and to support parenting efforts so that parents feel confident and competent.

TRANSITIONAL PERIOD

The transitional period involves two periods of reactivity separated by a sleep phase, called the first period of reactivity and the second period of reactivity. The characteristics of each period demonstrate the newborn's progression to independent functioning.

First Period of Reactivity

The first period of reactivity lasts for approximately 30 minutes after birth.

Characteristics

- The newborn's vital signs are as follows: rapid apical pulse rate that is irregular in rhythm. Respiratory rate (RR) as high as 80 breaths per minute, irregular, and possibly labored, with nasal flaring, expiratory grunting, and chest retractions. Color fluctuates from pale pink to cyanotic.

- Bowel sounds are usually absent, and the baby usually does not void or have a bowel movement during this period.
- The newborn has minimal amounts of mucus at this time, a rigorous cry, and strong suck reflex.

  Special tip: During this period, the newborn's eyes are open more than they will be again for days. It is an excellent time for the attachment process to begin because the newborn is able to maintain eye contact for long periods of time. It is a natural opportunity to initiate breast-feeding.

Care Needs Specific to First Period of Reactivity

1. Assess and monitor heart rate and respirations q30min for the first 4 hours after birth.
2. Keep baby warm (axillary or skin probe temperature between 36.5°C and 37°C [97.7°F–98.6°F]) with warmed blankets or overhead warming lights.
3. Place mother and baby together skin to skin to facilitate attachment.
4. Delay instillation of eye prophylactic for first hour to promote newborn–parent interaction.

Sleep Phase

The sleep phase begins about 30 minutes after the first period of reactivity and may last from a minute to 2–4 hours.

Characteristics

- As the baby moves into the sleep phase, the heart rate and respirations decrease. While asleep, the RR and the apical pulse rate return to baseline values.
- Skin color stabilizes; some acrocyanosis may be present. Bowel sounds become audible.

Care needs specific to sleep phase: The baby does not respond to external stimuli, but the mother and father can still enjoy holding and cuddling their baby.

Second Period of Reactivity

The second period of reactivity lasts about 4–6 hours.

Characteristics

- Baby has intense sensitivity to internal and environmental stimuli. Apical pulse ranges from 120–160 beats per minute. RR is 30–60 breaths per minute with periods of more rapid respirations, but respirations remain unlabored (no nasal flaring or retractions).
- Skin color fluctuates from pink or ruddy to mildly cyanotic with periods of mottling. Baby may be very active.
- Baby often voids and passes meconium during this period.
- Mucous secretions increase and the baby may gag on secretions. Sucking reflex is again strong, and baby may be very active.

Care Needs Specific to Second Period of Reactivity

1. Close observation of newborn for possible choking on the excessive mucus normally present. Use bulb syringe to remove mucus and teach parents how to use the bulb syringe.
2. Observe for any episode of apnea and drop in heart rate. Initiate methods of stimulation if needed (e.g., stroke baby's back, turn baby to side).
3. Assess baby's interest in feeding (sucking, rooting, and swallowing) and ability to feed (no choking or gagging during feeding, no vomiting of feeding in unchanged form).

Additional Assessments and Interventions in the Transitional Period

In these first few hours of life, the nurse will accomplish the following:

1. Monitor newborn vital signs. See Table 5–1 for summary of normal findings. (See Appendix E for additional information regarding selected newborn laboratory values.)
2. Weigh the newborn and measure length, head, and chest circumference (see Table 5–2 and Figure 5–1). To determine length, place the newborn flat on the

Table 5–1 Key Signs of Newborn Transition

Apical pulse: 120–160 beats per minute

    During sleep as low as 100 beats per minute; if crying, up to 180 beats per minute

    Apical pulse counted for 1 full minute

Respirations: 30–60 respirations per minute

    Predominantly diaphragmatic but synchronous with abdominal movements

    Brief periods of apnea (less than 15 sec), with no color or heart rate changes

Temperature

    Axillary: 36.4–37.2°C (97.5–99°F)

    Skin: 36–36.5°C (96.8–97.7°F)

Blood pressure: 90–60/50–40 mm Hg at birth; 100/50 mm Hg at day

Blood glucose: equal to or greater than 40 mg%

Hematocrit: less than 65%–70% central venous sample

Table 5–2 Newborn Weight and Measurements

Weight

    Average: 3,405 g (7 lb, 8 oz)

    Range: 2,500–4,000 g (5 lb, 8 oz, to 8 lb, 13 oz)

    Weight is influenced by racial origin and maternal age and size

    198 g (7 oz) growth per week for first 6 months

Length

    Average: 50 cm (20 in.)

    Range: 48–56 cm (18–22 in.)

Growth

    2 cm (1 in.) per month for first 6 months

Head Circumference

    Average: 32–37 cm (12$\frac{1}{2}$–14$\frac{1}{2}$ in.)

    Approximately 2 cm (about 1 in.) larger than chest circumference

Chest Circumference

    Average: 32 cm (12.5 in.)

    Range: 30–35 cm (12–14 in.)

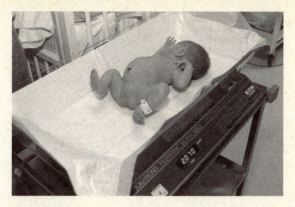

Figure 5–1 ■ Weighing of newborns. The scale is balanced with the protective pad in place.

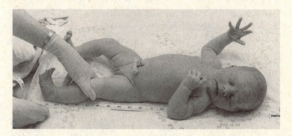

Figure 5–2 ■ Measuring the length of the newborn.

back with legs extended as much as possible. Hold the head still at the top of the measuring tape and gently stretch the legs downward toward the bottom of the tape (see Figure 5–2). To measure head circumference, place the tape over the most prominent part of the occiput and bring it around above the eyebrows (see Figure 5–3). The circumference of the head is approximately 2 cm greater than the circumference of the chest at birth.

To obtain chest circumference, place the tape measure at the lower edge of the scapulas and bring it around anteriorly over the nipple line.

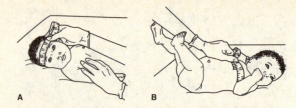

Figure 5–3 ■ Obtaining newborn measurements. **A,** Measuring the head circumference of the newborn. The tape is placed on the occiput and then brought around and placed just above the eyebrows. **B,** Measuring the chest circumference of the newborn. The tape is placed over the lower edge of the scapula and brought around to the front and placed over the nipple line.

3. Complete the gestational age assessment of the newborn during the first 4 hours of the newborn's life so that age-related problems can be identified. Clinical gestational age assessment tools have two components: external physical characteristics and neuromuscular status.

Physical characteristics (with the exception of sole creases) can be assessed over the first 24 hours. Neuromuscular development may be influenced by the newborn's unstable nervous system or labor and birth events. It can be assessed in the first 24 hours; however, if the findings drastically differ from the gestational age determined by looking at physical characteristics, the assessment may be repeated after 24 hours.

METHOD OF GESTATIONAL ASSESSMENT

Use Newborn Maturity Rating and Classification (Figure 5–4). Assess each of the factors listed and assign a score of 0–5 for each one. It is helpful to circle the results for each assessment.

Physical Maturity Characteristics

- **Skin** in the preterm newborn appears thin and transparent, with veins prominent over the abdomen early in gestation. As newborns approach term gestation, the

NEWBORN MATURITY RATING & CLASSIFICATION

ESTIMATION OF GESTATIONAL AGE BY MATURITY RATING
Symbols: X - 1st Exam   O - 2nd Exam

NEUROMUSCULAR MATURITY

	-1	0	1	2	3	4	5
Posture							
Square Window (wrist)	>90	90	60	45	30	0	
Arm Recoil		180	140–180	110–140	90–110	<90	
Popliteal Angle	180	160	140	120	100	90	<90
Scarf Sign							
Heel to Ear							

Gestation by Dates _ _ _ _ _ _ wks

Birth Date _ _ _ _ Hour _ _ _ _ am/pm

APGAR _ _ _ _ 1 min _ _ _ _ 5 min

MATURITY RATING

score	weeks
-10	20
-5	22
0	24
5	26
10	28
15	30
20	32
25	34
30	36
35	38
40	40
45	42
50	44

PHYSICAL MATURITY

Skin	sticky friable transparent	gelatinous red, translucent	smooth pink, visible veins	superficial peeling &/or rash, few veins	cracking pale areas rare veins	parchment deep cracking no vessels	leathery cracked wrinkled
Lanugo	none	sparse	abundant	thinning	bald areas	mostly bald	
Plantar Surface	heel-toe 40–50mm:-1 <40mm:-2	>50mm no crease	faint red marks	anterior transverse crease only	creases ant. 2/3	creases over entire sole	
Breast	imperceptible	barely perceptible	flat areola no bud	stippled areola 1–2mm bud	raised areola 3–4mm bud	full areola 5–10mm bud	
Eye/Ear	lids fused loosely:-1 tightly:-2	lids open pinna flat stays folded	sl. curved pinna; soft; slow recoil	well curved pinna; soft but ready recoil	formed & firm instant recoil	thick cartilage ear stiff	
Genitals male	scrotum flat, smooth	scrotum empty faint rugae	testes in upper canal rare rugae	testes descending few rugae	testes down good rugae	testes pendulous deep rugae	
Genitals female	clitoris prominent labia flat	prominent clitoris small labia minora	prominent clitoris enlarging minora	majora & minora equally prominent	majora large minora small	majora cover clitoris & minora	

SCORING SECTION

	1st Exam = X	2nd Exam = O
Estimating Gest Age by Maturity Rating	_ _ _ Weeks	_ _ _ Weeks
Time of Exam	Date _ _ _ _ Hour_ _ _ am/pm	Date _ _ _ _ Hour_ _ _ am/pm
Age at Exam	_ _ _ Hours	_ _ _ Hours
Signature of Examiner	_____ M.D.	_____ M.D.

Figure 5–4 ■ Newborn maturity rating and classification.

Source: From "New Ballard Score, Expanded to Include Extremely Premature Infants," by J. L. Ballard, J. C. Khoury, K. Wedig, L. Wang, B. L. Eilers-Walsmann, & R. Lipp, 1991, *Journal of Pediatrics, 119(3)*, 417.

skin appears opaque because of increased subcutaneous tissue. Disappearance of the protective vernix caseosa promotes skin desquamation (peeling), and this is commonly seen in postterm infants (infants of greater than 42 weeks' gestation).

- **Lanugo**, a fine hair covering, decreases as gestational age increases. The amount of lanugo is greatest at 28–30 weeks and then disappears, first from the face and then from the trunk and extremities.
- **Sole (plantar creases)** needs to be assessed within 12 hours of birth because afterward the skin of the foot begins drying and superficial creases disappear.

Development of sole creases begins at the top of the sole and proceeds downward toward the heel. Plantar creases vary with race. In newborns of African descent, sole creases may be less developed at term gestation.

- **Areola** is inspected and the breast bud tissue is gently palpated to determine the size. It is important to place your index and middle finger over this tissue and roll over the breast bud to estimate the size, rather than pinching the tissue, to avoid causing trauma. Another method of measuring involves placing a ruler just above the breast bud tissue for more accurate measurement. Most experienced nurses have completed the assessment often enough that they can estimate the size very accurately.

- **Ear form and cartilage** change throughout gestation. By 36 weeks some cartilage and slight incurving of the upper pinna are present, and the pinna springs back slowly when folded.

  To assess, observe ear form and then fold the pinna of the ear forward against the side of the head, release it, and observe the results.

- **Genitals** change in appearance during gestation because of the amount of subcutaneous fat present. **Female genitals** at 30–32 weeks have a prominent clitoris, and the labia majora are small and widely separated. At 36–40 weeks the labia nearly cover the clitoris, and at more than 40 weeks the labia majora completely cover the labia minora and clitoris. Complete the assessment by observation. **Male genitals** are evaluated for size of the scrotal sac, presence of rugae, and descent of the testes. Observe the size of the scrotal sac and the presence or absence of rugae. The scrotal sac can be gently palpated to determine descent of the testes.

Neuromuscular Maturity Characteristics

The neuromuscular maturity evaluation requires more manipulation and disturbances than the physical evaluation. It is best performed when the newborn has stabilized.

- **Resting posture** should be assessed while the baby lies undisturbed on a flat surface such as his or her bed.

- **Square window (wrist)** is elicited by flexing the baby's hand toward the ventral forearm until resistance is felt. The angle formed at the wrist is measured (by estimation and matching it against the angles on the scoring tool) (see Figure 5–5).

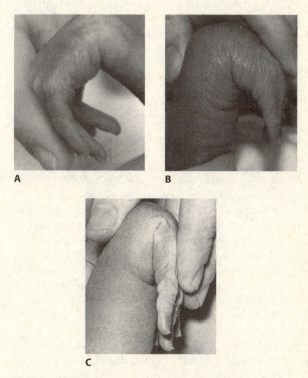

A

B

C

Figure 5–5 ■ Square window sign. **A,** This angle is 90 degrees and suggests an immature newborn of 28–32 weeks' gestation. (Score 0.) **B,** A 30-degree angle is commonly found from 39–40 weeks' gestation. (Score 2–3.) **C,** A 0-degree angle can occur from 40–42 weeks. (Score 4.)

Source: **C** is from *The Gestation Age of the Newborn*, by L. Dubowitz & V. Dubowitz, 1977, Menlo Park, CA: Addison-Wesley. Reprinted by permission of V. Dubowitz, MD, Hammersmith Hospital, London, England.

- **Arm recoil** is a test of flexion development. It is best evaluated after the first hour of life, when the baby has had time to recover from the stress of birth. To assess, place the newborn in a supine position (lying on the back), completely flex both elbows (by holding the newborn's hands and placing the hands up against the forearms), hold them in this position for about 5 seconds, and then release them. On release, the elbows of a full-term newborn form an angle of less than 90 degrees and rapidly recoil back to flexed position. The arms of a preterm newborn have slower recoil time and form greater than a 90-degree angle. Deep sleep state also decreases the arm recoil response. Assessment of arm recoil should be bilateral to rule out brachial palsy.

- **Popliteal angle** is determined with the newborn flat on his or her back. Flex the thigh on the newborn's abdomen and chest and place the index finger of your other hand behind the newborn's ankle to extend the lower leg until resistance is met. Then measure the angle formed. Results vary from no resistance in the very immature infant to an 80-degree angle in the term infant.

- **Scarf sign** is elicited by placing the newborn supine and drawing an arm across the chest toward the infant's opposite shoulder until resistance is met. (Newborns need to remain lying on their backs. The location of the elbow is then noted in relation to the midline of the chest) (see Figure 5–6). A preterm newborn's elbow will cross the midline of the chest, whereas a full-term infant's elbow will not cross midline.

- **Heel to ear** is performed by placing the baby in a supine position and, while stabilizing the hip on the bed, gently drawing the foot toward the ear on the same side until resistance is felt. Both the degree of knee extension and the proximity of the foot to the ear are assessed. In a very preterm newborn, the leg will remain straight and the foot will go to the ear or beyond. With advancing gestational age the newborn demonstrates increasing resistance to this maneuver. If the newborn was in a frank breech presentation, this

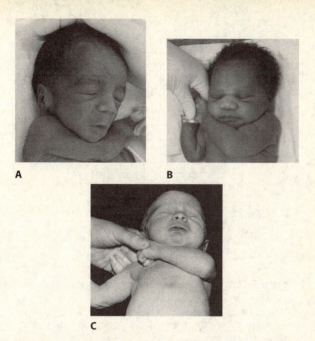

A **B**

C

Figure 5–6 ■ Scarf sign. **A,** No resistance is noted until after 30 weeks' gestation. The elbow moves readily past the midline. (Score 1.) **B,** The elbow is at midline at 36–40 weeks' gestation. (Score 2.) **C,** Beyond 40 weeks' gestation the elbow will not reach the midline. (Score 4.)

Source: **C** is from *The Gestation Age of the Newborn*, by L. Dubowitz & V. Dubowitz, 1977, Menlo Park, CA: Addison-Wesley. Reprinted by permission of V. Dubowitz, MD, Hammersmith Hospital, London, England.

assessment should be delayed until the legs are positioned more normally.

Gestational Age Scoring

All the individual scores are added and the total number is compared with the score on the Newborn Maturity Rating and Classification tool. A score of 35 equals 38 weeks, a score of 37 equals 39 weeks, and a score of 40 equals 40 weeks. The estimated gestational age is then plotted on

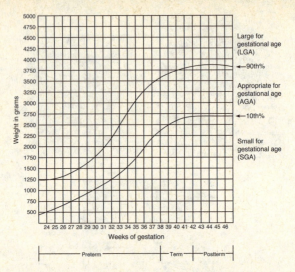

Figure 5–7 ■ Classification of newborns by birth weight and gestational age. The nurse places the newborn's birth weight and gestational age on the graph and classifies the newborn as large for gestational age (LGA), appropriate for gestational age (AGA), or small for gestational age (SGA).

Source: From "A Practical Classification of Newborn Infants by Weight and Gestational Age," by F. C. Battaglia & L. O. Lubchenco, 1967, *Journal of Pediatrics, 71,* 161.

a tool that classifies newborns by birth weight and gestational age (see Figure 5–7). Most newborns are appropriate for gestational age (AGA). A baby that is large for gestational age (LGA; growth above the 90th percentile) or small for gestational age (SGA; growth below the 10th percentile) may require additional assessment and intervention (for further discussion, see Chapter 6).

INITIAL NURSING INTERVENTIONS

- Administer erythromycin (Ilotycin) ointment (or tetracycline) into the newborn's eyes. This is a legally required prophylactic eye treatment for *Neisseria gonorrhoeae* and *Chlamydia* that may have infected the newborn

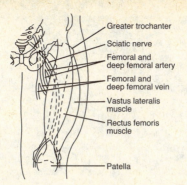

Figure 5–8 ■ Newborn injection sites. The middle third of the preferred site for intramuscular injection in the newborn.

during the birth process. Ilotycin has the advantage of being useful for treating both gonorrhea and *Chlamydia*; it is also less irritating to the newborn's eyes, which results in decreased incidence of swelling and discharge. (See Drug Guide: Erythromycin Ophthalmic Ointment [Ilotycin Ophthalmic], pp. 292–293.)

- Administer prophylactic dose of vitamin K. Vitamin K is given to prevent hemorrhage, which can occur because of low prothrombin levels in the first few days of life. (See Figure 5–8 for injection sites and Drug Guide: Vitamin K_1, Phytonadione [AquaMEPHYTON], pp. 310–311.)

- Assess glucose level. A drop of blood is obtained by heel stick and blood glucose is determined (see Figure 5–9). The glucose oxidase reagent strip or glucose oxidase analyzer should read greater than 40 mg/dL; a value less than 40 mg/dL needs to be followed up by drawing a central blood sample (drawn from a vein in the hand or antecubital space) for further laboratory evaluation. Treatment is begun if needed (see Chapter 6 for discussion of hypoglycemia). *Be alert for* hypoglycemia in high-risk babies such as SGA, infant of diabetic mother (IDM), AGA preterm, and any newborn who was stressed during labor and at birth. Outward signs

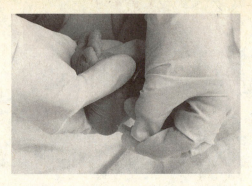

Figure 5–9 ■ Blood is obtained by a heel stick for a glucose test.

of hypoglycemia may include lethargy, jitteriness, poor feeding, vomiting, pallor, apnea, irregular respirations, and/or tremors.

• Maintain temperature through use of a controlled radiant warmer. A probe is placed on the newborn's abdomen just under the ribs or over the area of the liver. The probe indicates the newborn's temperature, and the radiant heater responds by becoming warmer or cooler. *Be alert for* newborns at risk for hypothermia (temperature less than 36.5°C [97.7°F]), including preterm, SGA, and any baby who was stressed at birth. If the newborn's temperature is 36.5°C (97.7°F) or below (axillary or skin probe temperature), rewarming is needed. Place the baby under a radiant warmer, undressing him or her so that the skin can be warmed. When the skin probe indicates that the desired temperature has been reached, recheck axillary temperature. The baby may be removed from the warmer; however, axillary temperature should be rechecked about every 30 minutes until the baby reaches desired temperature, then hourly until stable. Successful transition to extrauterine existence is documented by stabilization of vital signs and establishment of awake-sleep cycles and feeding, stooling, and voiding patterns. (See Procedures: Thermoregulation of the Newborn, pp. 356–359.)

POST-TRANSITIONAL NEWBORN NURSING CARE

Normal newborn care usually includes assessment of vital signs (axillary temperature, apical pulse, and respirations) every 6–8 hours, care of the umbilical stump per agency protocol, feeding on demand or at least every 3–4 hours, diapering as needed, and weighing once every 24 hours.

Physical Assessment

It is usually easier to proceed from head to toe; however, you need to assess axillary temperature, apical pulse, and respirations while the baby is quiet. Completing the assessment in the mother's room provides a wonderful opportunity for teaching, sharing, and role modeling for first-time mothers.

- **Skin color.** Inspect. Ensure skin color is appropriate for ethnic grouping. All healthy newborns have a pink tinge to their skin. Any evidence of acrocyanosis usually should have abated. Observe closely for signs of jaundice. Jaundice is first detectable on the face, the mucous membranes of the mouth, and the sclera. It is evaluated by blanching the tip of the nose, the forehead, the sternum, or the gum line. If jaundice is present, the area will appear yellowish immediately after blanching. Laboratory testing will verify the total bilirubin level. *Jaundice noted before 24 hours of age should be reported.* Jaundice requires additional assessment, evaluation, and then treatment as needed. The jaundice may be treated with phototherapy.

  Common variations: Milia may be present over the nose. A variety of markings may be present on the skin (see Table 5–3).

  Be alert for cyanosis; it requires immediate reassessment and treatment. Pallor may be associated with anemia, and

Table 5–3   Birthmarks

Type	Characteristics	Parent Teaching
Telangiectatic nevi (stork bites)	Pale pink or red flat dilated capillaries over eyelids, nose, and nape of neck	Seen more with crying. Blanch easily, fade by 2 years of age, no clinical significance.
Mongolian spots	Bluish-black or gray-blue macular areas over dorsal area and buttocks	Common in newborns of Asian, Hispanic, and African descent and other dark-skinned races. Gradually fade in first to second year of life. Mistaken for bruises—must document in newborn chart.
Nevus flammeus (port-wine stain)	Nonelevated, sharply outlined, red-to-purple dense area of capillaries, commonly on face; in black infants may appear as a purple-black stain	Does not fade with time or blanch as a rule. Can cover with opaque cosmetic cream. Suggestive of Sturge-Weber syndrome (involving 5th cranial nerve) if associated with neurologic problems.

ruddiness may indicate an elevated hematocrit (greater than 65%).

- **Head.** Palpate and observe fontanelles. The anterior fontanelle is the largest and is diamond shaped. The posterior fontanelle is triangular in shape. The sagittal suture (located on the top of the head, from front to back) is smooth and without ridges.

Common variations: Bulging of fontanelle (increased intracranial pressure), depressed fontanelle (dehydration), overriding of sagittal suture (molding), caput succedaneum (edema in tissues from trauma), cephalhematoma (bleeding into the periosteal space).

See Table 5–4.

Be alert for premature closing of both anterior and posterior sutures (craniosynostosis), which requires further assessment.

Table 5–4 Comparison of Cephalhematoma and Caput Succedaneum

Cephalhematoma

 Collection of blood between cranial (usually parietal) bone and periosteal membrane

 Does not cross suture lines

 Does not increase in size with crying

 Appears on first and second day

 Disappears after 2–3 weeks or may take months

Caput Succedaneum

 Collection of fluid, edematous swelling of the scalp

 Crosses suture lines

 Present at birth or shortly thereafter

 Reabsorbed within 12 hours or a few days after birth

- **Eyes.** Inspect eyes and lids. Eyes should be clear, without drainage or swelling of eyelids. Subconjunctival hemorrhage may be present. Sclera color tends to be white to bluish because of its relative thinness.

Common variations: Swelling of eyelid (birth trauma, reaction to eye prophylaxis).

Be alert for purulent drainage, an indication for further assessment for infection and treatment. A blue sclera is associated with osteogenesis imperfecta.

- **Ears.** Inspect outer ear. A full-term baby has incurving of the top two-thirds of the pinna. The top of the ear should be parallel to an imaginary line drawn from the inner canthus to the outer canthus of the eye and extended around toward the ear. Rotation of the ear should be in the midline and not tipped forward or backward.

Be alert for low-set ears, which may be associated with a variety of congenital problems.

- **Nose.** Inspect. Nares should be clear and without mucus. (Remember, newborns are obligatory nose breathers, so a stuffy nose has much greater implications for a newborn baby.)

Common variations: None.

Be alert for presence of nasal flaring. If present, assess RR, chest retractions, grunting, and skin color. A pulse-oximeter determination may provide further information (reading should be above 90%).

- **Mouth.** Check for asymmetric movement of the mouth. Inspect inside of mouth and palpate hard palate. Hard and soft palate should be intact (may visualize while the baby is crying or may palpate with an unpowdered gloved finger). (An opening indicates cleft palate.) Inspect gums for supernumerary (precocious) teeth (these teeth usually do not cause a problem but may loosen and fall out unexpectedly).

Common variations: Supernumerary (precocious) teeth and Epstein's pearls (small glistening white specks).

Be alert for an opening in the palate (cleft palate), which needs to be evaluated quickly. Presence of white patches on the mucous membranes that appear as milk deposits but cannot be wiped away with a 4 × 4 gauze pad may indicate thrush (*Candida albicans*). Excessive mucus may be associated with esophageal atresia. Asymmetric mouth movements when newborn cries may indicate transient nerve paralysis resulting from birth trauma.

- **Chest.** Inspect. Chest should be symmetric. Breasts may be flat or slightly enlarged (by the third day of life) because of the effects of maternal estrogen (this can last up to 2 weeks). Count RR over 1 minute (uncover baby and look at movement of chest or abdomen). See Table 5–1 for key signs of newborn transitions.

Common variations: Supernumerary (extra) nipple(s).

Be alert for retractions (intercostal or sternal). If they are present, assess RR and determine baby's need for oxygen.

- **Heart.** Auscultate. Apical pulse ranges from 120–160 beats per minute but may be as low as 100 beats per minute with sleep. Auscultate *apical rate for 1 full minute* when the newborn is asleep. Palpate brachial, radial, femoral, and pedal pulses. Compare brachial pulses bilaterally and with the femoral pulses.

Common variations: A transitory murmur may be heard for the first few hours of life.

Be alert for bradycardia (less than 100 beats per minute) or tachycardia (greater than 160 beats per minute).

- **Abdomen.** Inspect, auscultate, and palpate. Abdomen should be flat to slightly rounded (without distention), and bowel sounds should be heard in all quadrants. Umbilical stump is white and gelatinous with two umbilical arteries and one umbilical vein, should be drying, and have no redness, discharge, or bleeding.

Be alert for bleeding and/or purulent drainage from cord, which requires further assessment and treatment. Umbilical hernias are more common in infants of African descent.

- **Genitals.** Inspect. Genitals should be clearly differentiated. Both testes should be palpable in scrotum. Labia majora, labia minora, and clitoris size should be appropriate for gestational age.

Common variations: Pseudomenstruation (small amount of vaginal bleeding) in female infants due to maternal estrogen exposure; clear mucus from the vagina; vaginal skin tag. Smegma, a white cheeselike substance, found between the labia.

Be alert for urinary meatus on the underside of the penis (hypospadias). Scrotal discoloration and edema (hydrocele, testicular torsion).

- **Back.** Inspect. Back should be smooth, with no tufts of hair present over the lower back.

Common variations: Mongolian spot over lower back.

- **Hips.** Inspect and perform Ortolani's maneuver to rule out congenital dislocation of hips (hip dislocatability). Legs should be of equal length, and the skin folds on both right and left posterior thighs should be symmetric (see Figure 5–10). To do Ortolani's maneuver, place newborn on her or his back. Place the palm of your right hand on the newborn's left knee and extend your index and middle finger toward the hip. Your fingertips should be on the top of the greater trochanter.

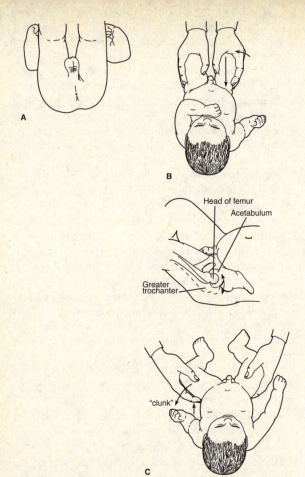

Figure 5–10 ■ **A,** Congenitally dislocated right hip in a young infant as seen on gross inspection. **B,** Barlow's (dislocation) maneuver. Baby's thigh is grasped and adducted with gentle downward pressure. Dislocation is palpable as femoral head slips out of acetabulum. **C,** Ortolani's maneuver puts downward pressure on the hip and then inward rotation. If the hip is dislocated, this forces the femoral head over the acetabular rim with a noticeable "clunk."

Source: From *Recognizable Patterns of Human Deformation*, by D. W. Smith, 1981, Philadelphia: Saunders.

Place your left hand in the same manner. With hips and knees flexed at a 90-degree angle, lift thigh to bring femoral head toward the acetabulum and apply gentle abduction. Feel for a "clunk" under your fingertips. If a clunk is felt, notify baby's care provider. The baby will most likely be placed in a Pavlik harness or abduction splint to keep the hip abducted.

- **Extremities.** Inspect. All extremities should be symmetric and move equally. Count digits on hands and feet; inspect palmar creases and check for clubfoot. Note any webbing (syndactyly).

Common variations: None.

Be alert for asymmetric movement or no movement of an extremity, which needs to be reported and assessed further.

- **Anus.** Inspect. Anus is patent and without fissures. Meconium passes within 24–48 hours after birth.

Common variations: None.

Be alert for failure to pass first meconium stool that may indicate imperforate anus, rectal atresia, or meconium ileus.

- **Elimination.** Note newborn record. Newborn should void within 24 hours and have a bowel movement within 48 hours after birth. After that, most babies have 6–8 wet diapers a day and may stool at least once a day. Breast-fed babies tend to have more frequent stools.

Common variations: None.

Be alert if baby does not void within 24 hours. Assess amount of fluid taken in and urethral opening. If no stool, assess abdomen for distention and bowel sounds. Diarrhea stools can be very serious for the newborn. Observe stool characteristics closely and test the stool for occult blood (Hematest) and sugar loss (Clinitest or other glucose testing).

- **Behavioral.** Observe. Baby quiets to soothing, cuddling, or wrapping and moves through all sleep-awake states. When held in front of parent or caregiver, baby will turn head toward sound.

Common variations: None.

Be alert for excessive crying, fretfulness, and inability to quiet self, which may be associated with drug withdrawal in the newborn.

Tip: Completing the behavioral assessment in the mother's room provides a wonderful opportunity for learning about the individual baby's cues and personality.

Assessment of Reflexes

At some point during the time you spend with this newborn, assess normal newborn reflexes.

- **Moro.** Elicited by startling the newborn with a loud noise or sudden movement. Newborn straightens arms and hands out while flexing knees. The arms then return to the chest as in an embrace. The fingers spread, forming a C, and the infant may cry.
- **Grasp.** Elicited by stimulating the newborn's palm with a finger or object. The newborn grasps and holds the object or finger firmly enough to be lifted momentarily from the crib.
- **Rooting.** Elicited when the side of the newborn's mouth or cheek is touched. In response, the newborn turns toward that side and opens the lips to suck.

Documentation of Assessment Findings and Care

Assessment findings may be recorded on computer charting systems, on newborn flow sheets, or in narrative notes. A narrative note might be recorded as follows:

Anterior fontanelle soft and flat, posterior fontanelle palpated closed at this time, some molding present with overriding of sagittal suture, caput succedaneum over posterior aspect of head. Eyes clear and without discharge or swelling. Nares clear without flaring or discharge. Mouth clear, and palate intact. Chest movements symmetrical without retractions, apical pulse 134, regular, and no murmurs. Abdomen soft and nondistended. Bowel sounds × 4. Baby has had a meconium and transitional stool. Umbilical stump drying and without redness or discharge. No redness or discharge noted on genitalia. Perineal area cleansed and A and D ointment applied. Back clear. Moves all extremities equally. No hip click. Palmar creases normal. Skin color appropriate to ethnic group and without cyanosis. Soothes with cuddling and rocking. M. Chin, RNC

ADDITIONAL ASPECTS OF NEWBORN DAILY CARE

- **Suctioning.** Achieved by compressing the bulb syringe; the tip is placed in the nostril. Make sure to take care not to occlude the passageway. The bulb is permitted to re-expand slowly by releasing the compression on the bulb. The bulb syringe is removed from the nostril, and drainage is then compressed out of the bulb onto a tissue. The bulb syringe may also be inserted into the side of the mouth, and the compression of the bulb is then slowly released. The bulb should be withdrawn and the contents expelled onto a paper towel or cloth. The bulb is then recompressed and placed into the other side of the mouth if needed. Avoid suctioning the roof of the mouth and back of throat. It is best to have the bulb available at all times for the newborn. It is important to teach the parents the use of the bulb at their first contact with the baby. Some parents are frightened of the bulb, and it helps for them to actually hold it and compress it. When choking occurs, the baby may be picked up and held with the head slightly down and the mouth to the side to facilitate the drainage of mucus. It can be frightening to deal with a choking baby.

- **Sleep and activity.** Place the baby on her or his back for sleeping to reduce incidence of sudden infant death syndrome. This serves to educate parents regarding infant positioning. The baby can be placed on her or his side initially if copious or thick secretions exist or if the baby is regurgitating feedings; but explain to family the reason for the alternative positioning. It is important to assist parents as they develop sensitivity to their infant's communication signals and rhythms of activity and sleep.

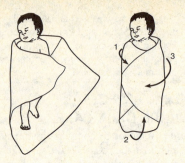

Figure 5–11 ▧ Steps used for swaddling a baby.

- **Swaddling.** The newborn seems to be comforted by being wrapped snugly in blankets (see Figure 5–11).
- **Holding.** To pick up the newborn, slide one hand up under the shoulders and neck to the head and the other hand under the buttocks or between the legs. The baby can now be picked up and placed upon your shoulder or cradled in the crook of your arm. (Sometimes it is easier to place the baby against your shoulder first, get settled, and then change the baby to the crook of your arm. If you are right handed, you will tend to be most comfortable cradling the baby in your left arm. Remember to teach new parents this technique.) The baby may also be held in a football hold.
- **Circumcision care.** Before the procedure, the parents need to validate that they understand the procedure and sign an informed consent form. Some form of analgesia is recommended: EMLA Cream (lidocaine 2.5% and prilocaine 2.5%), dorsal penile nerve block, or subcutaneous ring block. After the circumcision, the penis needs to be assessed for bleeding and infection. If a clamp is used, petroleum ointment is applied at each diaper change to provide protection to the skin and keep the penis from sticking to the diaper. If a Plastibell is used, the remaining plastic ring protects the penis and petroleum ointment may be used after Plastibell falls

off. Other than cleansing by letting warm water softly rinse over the penis to clear away urine and patting it dry, no other care is required. The Plastibell usually falls off by itself. If it is still in place after 8 days, the parents need to contact their care provider.

Comfort measures during circumcision include lightly stroking the baby's head, providing a sucrose pacifier, and talking to baby. Immediately after the circumcision, comfort measures may include wrapping the baby in soft blankets and rocking, walking with the baby, using a pacifier, feeding after initial crying has abated, singing, gently rubbing the back, talking to the baby, and using therapeutic touch (use short, light, feathery strokes for a short period of time).

- **Newborn screening tests.** Before the newborn's discharge, blood needs to be obtained by heel stick for phenylketonuria and congenital hypothyroidism testing. The newborn needs to be at least 24 hours old for a valid test. A second phenylketonuria test should be done by 2 weeks of age if the first test was done before 24 hours of age. It is important to stress the need for the second test with the parents, and that it is usually done on an outpatient basis. Newborn screening may also be done for cystic fibrosis, galactosemia, congenital adrenal hyperplasia, biotinidase deficiency, sickle cell trait, and hemoglobinopathies. The Expanded Newborn Screening program allows parents to have their babies screened for more than 20 disorders. Universal newborn hearing screening is recommended before discharge in all hospitals providing birthing services.

- **Recombinant hepatitis B vaccine.** Universal hepatitis B vaccination for all infants, regardless of maternal hepatitis B surface antigen status, is currently recommended by the American Academy of Pediatrics (AAP) Committee on Fetus and Newborn & American College of Obstetricians and Gynecologists (ACOG) Committee on Obstetrics (2007). Infants born to hepatitis B surface antigen-positive mothers should

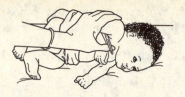

Figure 5–12 ■ The axillary temperature should be taken for 3 minutes. The newborn's arm should be tightly but gently pressed against the thermometer and the newborn's side.

receive hepatitis B vaccine and hepatitis B immune globulin (HBIG). (See Drug Guide: Hepatitis B Vaccine [Energix-B, Recombivax HB], pp. 293–294.)

PARENT EDUCATION

Provide information as needed on the following topics:

1. **Axillary temperature.** Place the thermometer in the baby's right or left axilla. The thermometer needs to be in contact with skin on all sides (see Figure 5–12). Hold the thermometer in place for 3 minutes unless an electronic thermometer is used. It is important to keep your hand on the thermometer at all times to ensure correct placement and prevent an accident. After reading the temperature, cleanse the thermometer by rinsing in cool water and wiping with a soft towel. Review normal range of temperature (axillary: 36.5–37.0°C [97.7–98.6°F]).

   Teaching tip: Ask parents what type of thermometer they will be using and plan your teaching to that specific type. This may be done in the birthing center and reinforced in the home during a home visit (see Chapter 9).

2. **Diapering with reusable cloth diapers.** Many diaper-folding methods are available, as well as diaper wraps that allow the diaper to be placed inside a Velcro-fastened wrapper (see Figure 5–13). Hand-washing before and after changing the diaper is essential.

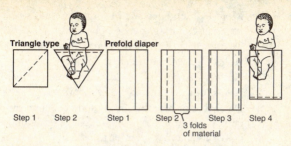

Triangle type   **Prefold diaper**

Step 1   Step 2   Step 1   Step 2   Step 3   Step 4
3 folds
of material

Figure 5–13 ■ Two methods of using cloth diapers.

3. **Diapering with single-use paper diapers.** The baby is placed on the diaper, the front is pulled up toward the navel, and the sides are brought forward and attached by a sticky tab to the front of the diaper. Care needs to be taken to fold the diaper below the level of the umbilicus for the first 7–10 days. In addition, soiled diapers should not be left in open waste containers. Hand-washing before and after changing the diaper is essential.

4. **Car safety.** It is mandatory that newborns go home in a rear-facing car seat until the baby is 1 year old or weighs 20 pounds (9.09 kg) (American Academy of Pediatrics, 2008). Parents should be knowledgeable about the benefits of child safety seat use and proper installation.

5. **When to call a healthcare provider.** The parents should call their healthcare provider if any of the following conditions occur:

   • Axillary temperature of greater than 38°C (100.4°F) or less than 36.6°C (97.8°F)
   • Continued rise in temperature
   • Cyanosis (bluish discoloration of skin) with or without a feeding
   • Absence of breathing longer than 20 seconds
   • Increasing jaundice (yellow tone) of the skin
   • Refusal of two feedings in a row

- More than one episode of forceful vomiting or frequent vomiting (over 6 hours)
- Two consecutive green, watery stools or black stools or increased frequency of stools
- No wet diapers for 18–24 hours or fewer than 6–8 wet diapers per day after 4 days of age
- Discharge or bleeding from umbilical cord, circumcision, or any opening (except vaginal mucus or pseudomenstruation)
- Pustules, rashes, or blisters other than normal newborn rash
- Inconsolable infant (quieting techniques are not effective) or continuous high-pitched cry
- Lethargy (listlessness), difficulty in awakening baby
- Development of eye drainage

REFERENCES

American Academy of Pediatrics (AAP). (2008). Car safety seats: A guide for families 2008. Retrieved April 20, 2008, from www.aap.org/family/carseatguide.

American Academy of Pediatrics (AAP), Committee on Fetus and Newborn & American College of Obstetricians and Gynecologists (ACOG) Committee on Obstetrics. (2007). *Guidelines for perinatal care* (6th ed.). Evanston, IL: Author.

6   THE AT-RISK NEWBORN

HYPOGLYCEMIA

- Condition of abnormally low levels of serum glucose. It can be defined as a blood glucose level below 40 mg/dL at any time after birth for all newborns or a glucose oxidase reagent strip with reflectance meter reading below 40 mg/dL when corroborated by a blood glucose test.
- In clinical practice, an infant with a plasma glucose level less than 40 mg/dL requires intervention. Also, plasma glucose values less than 20–25 mg/dL should be treated with parenteral glucose, regardless of the age or gestation to raise plasma glucose to greater than 45 mg/dL.
- Presentation of symptoms and blood glucose levels vary greatly with each baby. Symptoms usually occur at less than 40 mg/dL. Clinical manifestations vary greatly but can include tremors or jittery movements, irritability, lethargy or hypotonia, irregular respirations, apnea, cyanosis, pallor, refusal to suck or poor feeding, high-pitched or weak cry, hypothermia, diaphoresis, or neonatal seizure activity. When left untreated, hypoglycemia may cause neurodevelopmental outcomes.

Management of Hypoglycemia

- For at-risk infants who have not yet had a low blood sugar test, an oral feeding of formula or early breast-feeding is given with a follow-up blood glucose test within 30–60 minutes after feeding. If the baby cannot take formula or breast milk, a 5%–10% glucose intravenous (IV) infusion is ordered to prevent hypoglycemia. For symptomatic acute hypoglycemia, a bolus dose of D10W IV at a rate of 1–2 mL/kg is given, followed by 5%–10% glucose infusion.

- Intravenous glucose solution should be calculated based on body weight and fluid requirements and correlated with blood glucose tests to determine the adequacy of the infusion treatment.
- Administration of corticosteroid may be used for prolonged cases of hypoglycemia.

Nursing Assessments for Hypoglycemia

- Assess newborn and record for any risk factors.
  Be alert for special gestational newborns, such as premature, small for gestational age (SGA), and infant of diabetic mother (IDM) infants, and newborns with problems of asphyxia, cold stress, sepsis, or polycythemia. Also, maternal epidural anesthesia can alter maternal-fetal glucose homeostasis.
- Assess blood glucose reagent strip (see Procedures: Performing a Heel Stick on a Newborn, pp. 335–338). Newer techniques, such as using a glucose oxidase analyzer or an optical bedside glucose analyzer, are more reliable for bedside screening because interpreting the color is not as subjective. Infants in at-risk groups should be monitored within 30–60 minutes after birth and before feedings or whenever there are abnormal clinical manifestations. Assess IDMs within 30 minutes of birth. Once at-risk infant's blood sugar is stable, glucose testing every 2–4 hours (or per agency protocol), or before feedings, adequately monitors glucose levels.
  Note: Whole blood glucose concentrations are 10%–15% lower than plasma glucose concentrations.
- Assess all newborns for symptoms of hypoglycemia.

Sample Nursing Diagnoses

- *Acute pain* related to multiple heel sticks for glucose monitoring

- *Altered nutrition: less than body requirements* related to increased glucose use secondary to physiologic stresses
- *Ineffective family coping* related to fear over infant's condition

Nursing Interventions for Hypoglycemia

- Based on agency glucose testing protocol, provide early feedings of breast milk or formula for infants at risk for hypoglycemia.
- Obtain glucose oxidase reagent strip or optical bedside glucose analyzer reading per agency protocol. If less than 40 mg/dL, obtain STAT blood glucose per venous stick by lab. Then provide breast-feeding or formula (about 1 oz) to infant. Recheck glucose oxidase reagent strip or optical bedside glucose analyzer reading in 30–60 minutes. Obtain blood glucose levels q4–8h minimum.

  Note: If initial glucose oxidase reagent strip or optical bedside glucose analyzer reading is less than 20 mg/dL, obtain STAT blood glucose and start IV glucose therapy.

  Clinical Tip: Blood samples for the lab should be placed on ice and analyzed within 30 minutes of drawing to prevent the red blood cells (RBCs) from continuing to metabolize glucose.

- If IV therapy is ordered by the physician or indicated by your agency protocol
  1. Start 5%–10% dextrose and water IV on infusion pump and continue glucose infusion as per protocol.
  2. Administer infusion in peripheral vein of upper extremity to avoid lower extremity varicosities and potential tissue necrosis if IV infiltrates.
  3. Monitor titration of IV glucose during transition to oral glucose intake.
- Provide comfort measures to decrease crying and to ensure rest and maintain the optimal thermal environment specific for each newborn to reduce activity and glucose consumption. Nonnutritive sucking may lower activity levels and conserve baby's energy levels.

- Assist parents to identify feelings and concerns about baby's condition. Encourage and allow for maximum contact between parents and their baby.
- Review the following critical aspects of the care you have provided:
  1. Did I identify the baby's risk for hypoglycemia early in the baby's care?
  2. Have I been alert for the early signs of hypoglycemia?
  3. Have I monitored the blood glucose levels carefully and instituted care per agency protocol promptly?

Sample Nurse's Charting

0625 am T 97.7°F, P 150, R 35. Ant. fontanelle soft & flat. Breath sounds equal bilaterally, slight substernal retractions. Abdomen soft and nondistended. Hypoactive bowel sounds. Fine tremors of arms and hands. Glucose reagent strips less than 40 mg/dL. Poor suck, took 25 mL of 5% G/W with difficulty. STAT lab blood glucose pending. Baby placed under radiant warmer to stabilize temperature. Dr. Rich notified of glucose level. M. Chin, RNC

Evaluation

- Newborn's glucose level is stable at greater than 40 mg/dL, and the baby is symptom free.
- Newborn is free from further complications.

COLD STRESS

- Cold stress is excessive heat loss resulting in the use compensatory mechanisms (such as increased respirations, nonshivering thermogenesis, and use of brown fat stores) to maintain core body temperature. When babies become chilled, they increase their oxygen consumption and use of glucose for physiologic processes.
- Complications that occur because of this alteration in metabolic processes are respiratory distress, respiratory and metabolic acidosis, hypoglycemia, and jaundice.
- Premature, SGA, hypoxic, hypoglycemic, and central nervous system (CNS) depressed newborns are at

higher risk for becoming hypothermic and suffer the consequences.

Management of Cold Stress

Initially, clinical management is directed to prevention and then to the management required by the specific complication.

Nursing Assessments for Hypothermia

- Assess newborn temperature, using either axillary or skin probe method. Be alert for a drop in skin temperature (it drops before core temperature), which may be an early indicator of cold stress.

  Tip: Axillary temperature can be misleading because of the nearness to brown fat, which can increase heat production.

- Assess for additional signs of hypothermia: shallow, irregular respirations; retractions; diminished reflexes; bradycardia; oliguria; and lethargy.
- Assess for complications such as hyperbilirubinemia, hypoglycemia (blood glucose level less than 40 mg/dL), and respiratory distress.

Sample Nursing Diagnoses

- *Hypothermia* related to exposure to cold environment, trauma, illness, or inability to shiver
- *Ineffective thermoregulation* related to immaturity

Nursing Interventions for Hypothermia

- Institute measures to prevent heat loss due to radiation, evaporation, convection, and conduction. Measures include the following: dry off baby immediately and remove wet linen after birth; place baby on prewarmed bed under radiant heat source for all care and procedures; cover scales before weighing; warm stethoscope bell prior to auscultation; keep beds away from drafts and air vents; use warmed, humidified oxygen; warm IV fluids before infusion; keep baby wrapped when not skin to skin, cover head with stockinette hat, or place under radiant heat source with temperature probe in place; turn up thermostat in birthing area before birth; do not place warmer bed near windows or outside walls; use heated incubator for transport.

- If baby is chilled, rewarm slowly to prevent apnea (see Procedures: Thermoregulation of the Newborn, pp. 356–359).
- Monitor blood glucose levels for signs of hypoglycemia and arterial blood gases for signs of respiratory distress.
- Carry out care needed by newborns placed under phototherapy to maintain stable temperature. (See Management of Jaundice in this chapter.)
- Instruct parents about causes of temperature fluctuation, infant's current status, heat conservation methods, and temperature stabilization methods.
- Determine that parents understand ways to minimize heat loss and know how to obtain their newborn's temperature.
- Review the following critical aspects of the care you have provided:
  1. Have I provided for sufficient warmth during all procedures and care activities? During baths? During IV starts or blood work?
  2. Have I been alert for any signs of hypoglycemia, hyperbilirubinemia, or respiratory distress?
  3. Have I provided support and comfort to the baby?
  4. Have I kept the parents informed?

Evaluation

- Baby is maintained in a neutral thermal environment.
- Parents understand the importance of preventing heat loss and methods to prevent complications of hypothermia.

RESPIRATORY DISTRESS SYNDROME (RDS)

Respiratory distress syndrome (RDS) is a condition associated with prematurity and any factor resulting in a deficiency of functioning lung surfactant, such as a diabetic mother or hypoxia. Clinical manifestations may present at birth or within a few hours after birth. Clinical manifestations are tachypnea, expiratory grunting, nasal flaring on inspiration, subcostal or intercostal retractions, pallor and cyanosis, apnea, labored breathing, increasing need for oxygen, and hypotonus. The chest X-ray shows diffuse reticulogranular density bilaterally, with portions of the air-filled tracheobronchial tree (air bronchogram) outlined by the opaque lungs. RDS usually resolves over 7–10 days unless surfactant replacement therapy has been used.

Management of Respiratory Distress Syndrome

Supportive management involves oxygen administration, ventilation therapy, blood gas monitoring, transcutaneous oxygen and carbon dioxide monitoring or pulse oximeter methods, and correction of acid–base imbalance. Ventilatory therapy is aimed at preventing hypoventilation and hypoxia. The degree of ventilatory support needed ranges from increasing oxygen concentration and using continuous positive airway pressure (CPAP) to intubation and full mechanical ventilation. Surfactant-replacement therapy has been shown to improve oxygenation rapidly and decrease the need for ventilatory support. Surfactant-replacement therapy must be administered by specially trained personnel.

Nursing Assessment for Respiratory Distress Syndrome

- Assess newborn for any risk factors. Be alert for premature infants and any infant suspected of hypoxia in utero or soon after birth.
- Assess newborn's respiratory effort. Note chest wall movement, respiratory effort (grunting, nasal flaring, substernal or intercostal retractions), and color (cyanosis, pallor, duskiness) of skin and mucous membranes; auscultate lung for bilateral air entry.

Tip: At about 48–72 hours (if no surfactant-replacement therapy is given), when the alveoli begin to open up, watch the chest movement carefully, because the infant is at greatest risk for pneumothorax at this time.

- Assess need for increased oxygen and assisted ventilation measures.

  Note: Normal Pao_2: 50–70 mm Hg, $Paco_2$: 35–45 mm Hg, and pH 7.35–7.45. Monitor blood pressure (average for term infant, 90/50; preterm infant, 64/39).

- Assess intake and output (I&O) and electrolytes. Increased labored breathing (work of breathing) causes an increase in insensible water losses.

  Tip: As the lungs open up, there is usually an increase in voiding (as determined by weighing diapers), because more fluid moves into the bloodstream to be excreted by the kidneys.

- Assess for signs of infection: temperature instability, lethargy, poor feeding, and hypotonia.

Sample Nursing Diagnoses

- *Impaired gas exchange* related to inadequate lung surfactant
- *Risk for infection* related to invasive procedures

Nursing Interventions for Respiratory Distress Syndrome

- Administer warmed, humidified oxygen by designated route: oxygen hood, bag and mask, or intubation (Figure 6–1).
- Alter oxygen concentrations by 5%–10% increments or per order to maintain adequate Pao_2 levels. Obtain blood gas levels after any significant change in oxygen concentration.
- Obtain arterial blood gases per order. Maintain stable environment before blood gas studies (do not suction, change oxygen levels or ventilator settings, or disturb baby).

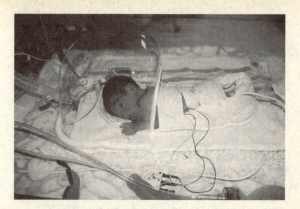

Figure 6–1 ■ Infant in oxygen hood.

- Suction as necessary. Secretions are sparse until second or third day, when the lungs start opening up. Watch transcutaneous oxygen monitor or pulse oximeter for desaturation during procedure.
- Check and calibrate all monitoring and measuring devices every 8 hours.
- Maintain patency of IVs via infusion pumps.
- Maintain a neutral thermal environment. Temperature instability increases oxygen consumption and metabolic acidosis.
- Administer medications per order: antibiotics, diuretics, sedatives, and analgesics. Fentanyl and morphine are used for their analgesic and sedative effects. The use of pancuronium (Pavulon) for muscle relaxation is controversial.
- Careful hand-washing, use of gloves during procedures, and attention to infection control are essential.
- Provide time to answer parents' questions about the baby's status and the equipment used and to give emotional support. Explain developmental supportive care to the parents.
- Record and report all clinical observations.

Evaluation

- The risk of RDS is promptly identified, and early intervention is initiated.
- The newborn is free of respiratory distress and metabolic alterations.
- The parents verbalize their concerns about their baby's health problem and survival and understand the rationale behind management of their newborn.

SPECIAL NEWBORNS AND THEIR ASSOCIATED CLINICAL PROBLEMS
Small for Gestational Age (SGA)/ Intrauterine Growth Restriction (IUGR)

Physical Characteristics

Large-appearing head in proportion to chest and abdomen
Loose, dry skin
Scarcity of subcutaneous fat, with emaciated appearance
Long, thin appearance
Sunken abdomen
Sparse scalp hair
Anterior fontanelle may be depressed May have vigorous cry and appears alert Birth weight below 10th percentile

Clinical Problems

1. **Asphyxia.** Chronic hypoxia in utero leaves little reserve to withstand the demands of labor and birth. Thus, intrauterine asphyxia occurs, with its potential systemic problems.

2. **Aspiration syndrome.** Gasping secondary to in utero hypoxia can cause aspiration of amniotic fluid into the lower airways or can lead to relaxation of the anal sphincter with passage of meconium. This results in meconium aspiration with first breaths after birth.

Physical Characteristics	Clinical Problems

Physical Characteristics

Clinical Problems

3. **Hypothermia.** Decreased ability to conserve heat results from diminished subcutaneous fat (used for survival in utero), depletion of brown fat in utero, and large surface area.

   The surface area is diminished somewhat because of the flexed position assumed by the small for gestational age infant. (See Cold Stress discussed earlier in this chapter.)

4. **Hypoglycemia.** High metabolic rate (secondary to heat loss), poor liver glycogen stores, and inhibited gluconeogenesis lead to low blood sugar levels. (See Hypoglycemia discussed earlier in this chapter.)

5. **Polycythemia.** A physiologic response to in utero chronic hypoxic stress increases the number of red blood cells. Polycythemia may contribute to hypoglycemia.

6. **Congenital malformations.** Secondary to cellular hypoplasia and impaired mitotic activity.

Infant of Diabetic Mother (IDM)

Physical Characteristics

Appears large and fat
Cushingoid facial (round
face) and neck features
Overall ruddiness Has
enlarged liver, spleen,
and heart

Clinical Problems

1. **Hypoglycemia.** After birth,
   the most common problem
   of an IDM is hypoglycemia.
   Even though the high maternal blood supply is lost, this
   newborn continues to produce
   high levels of insulin, which
   deplete the blood glucose
   within hours after birth.
   IDMs also have less ability
   to release glucagon and
   catecholamines, which
   normally stimulate glucagon
   breakdown and glucose
   release. (See Hypoglycemia
   discussed earlier in this
   chapter.)

2. **Hypocalcemia.** Associated
   with prematurity, hyper-
   phosphatemia, or asphyxia.

3. **Hyperbilirubinemia.** This
   condition may be seen at
   48–72 hours after birth. It
   may be caused by slightly
   decreased extracellular fluid
   volume, which increases
   the hematocrit level.
   Cephalhematoma, or
   enclosed hemorrhages,
   resulting from complicated
   vaginal birth may also cause
   hyperbilirubinemia. There
   may also be an increase
   in the rate of bilirubin

Physical Characteristics	Clinical Problems

production in the presence of polycythemia. (See Jaundice discussed later in this chapter.)

4. **Polycythemia.** This condition may be caused by the decreased extracellular volume. In IDMs, hemoglobin $A1_c$ binds oxygen, which decreases the oxygen available to the fetal tissues. This tissue hypoxia stimulates increased erythropoietin production, which increases the hematocrit level. (See Polycythemia discussed later in this chapter.)

5. **Birth trauma.** Secondary to macrosomia, such as fractures of the clavicle, facial nerve paralysis, Erb's paralysis, and diaphragmatic paralysis.

6. **Respiratory distress.** This complication occurs especially in newborns of White's classes A–C diabetic mothers. The composition of the phospholipids themselves is altered in the lungs of IDMs. (See Respiratory Distress Syndrome discussed earlier in this chapter.)

IDM, infant of diabetic mother.

Preterm Infant

Physical Characteristics

Color—usually pink or ruddy but may be acrocyanotic; observe for cyanosis, jaundice, pallor, or plethora

Skin—reddened, translucent, blood vessels readily apparent, lack of subcutaneous fat

Lanugo—plentiful, widely distributed

Head size—appears large in relation to body

Skull—bones pliable, fontanelle smooth and flat

Ears—minimal cartilage, pliable, folded over

Nails—soft, short

Genitals—small; testes may not be descended

Resting position—flaccid, froglike

Cry—weak, feeble

Reflexes—poor sucking, swallowing, and gagging

Activity—jerky, generalized movements (seizure activity is abnormal)

Clinical Problems

1. **Apnea of prematurity**. Cessation of breathing for 20 seconds or longer or for less than 20 seconds when associated with cyanosis and bradycardia. It is thought to be primarily a result of neuronal immaturity, a factor that contributes to the tendency for irregular breathing patterns in preterm infants. Gastroesophageal reflux (GER) has been implicated in the production of apnea (causing laryngospasm).

2. **Patent ductus arteriosus.** Failure of ductus arteriosus to close because of decreased pulmonary arteriole musculature and hypoxemia.

3. **Respiratory distress syndrome (RDS).** Respiratory distress results from inadequate surfactant production. (See Respiratory Distress Syndrome discussed earlier in this chapter.)

4. **Intraventricular hemorrhage.** Up to 35 weeks' gestation, the preterm infant's brain ventricles are lined by the germinal matrix, which is highly susceptible to hypoxic

Clinical Problems

events. The germinal matrix is very vascular, and these blood vessels rupture in the presence of hypoxia.

5. **Hypoglycemia.** The preterm infant's decreased brown fat and glycogen stores and increased metabolic needs predispose this infant to hypoglycemia. (See Hypoglycemia and Cold Stress discussed earlier in this chapter.)

6. **Anemia of prematurity.** The preterm infant is at risk for anemia because of the rapid rate of growth required, shorter red blood cell life, excessive blood sampling, decreased iron stores, and deficiency of vitamin E.

7. **Hyperbilirubinemia.** Immature hepatic enzymatic function decreases conjugation of bilirubin, resulting in increased bilirubin levels. (See Jaundice discussed later in this chapter.)

8. **Infection.** The preterm infant is more susceptible to infection than the term infant. Most of the newborn's immunity is acquired in the last trimester. Therefore, the preterm infant has decreased antibodies available for protection.

Post-Term Infant

Physical Characteristics

Generally has normal size skull, but small body makes skull look large

Dry, cracked skin

Nails extending beyond fingertips

Profuse scalp hair

Subcutaneous fat layers depleted, leaving skin loose and giving an "old person" appearance

Long and thin body contour

Absent vernix

Often meconium staining (golden yellow to green) of skin, nails, and cord

May have an alert, wide-eyed appearance symptomatic of chronic intrauterine hypoxia

Clinical Problems

1. **Hypoglycemia.** Nutritional deprivation and resultant depleted glycogen stores. (See Hypoglycemia discussed earlier in this chapter.)

2. **Meconium aspiration.** Response to hypoxia in utero.

3. **Polycythemia.** Due to increased production of red blood cells in response to hypoxia. (See Polycythemia discussed later in this chapter.)

4. **Congenital anomalies of unknown cause.**

5. **Seizure.** Due to hypoxic insult.

6. **Cold stress.** Due to loss or poor development of subcutaneous fat. (See Cold Stress discussed earlier in this chapter.)

HEMATOLOGIC PROBLEMS OF THE NEWBORN

Anemia

Term (hemoglobin [Hgb] less than 14 g/dL). Preterm (Hgb less than 13 g/dL). Most common causes are blood loss, hemolysis/erythrocyte destruction, and impaired RBC/erythrocyte production.

Characteristics

Pale, 3-second capillary refill, decreased pulses, slow weight gain in first months of life. Tachycardia may be present.

Critical Nursing Management

Preventive: Term baby: Provide iron-fortified formula or iron supplementation.

Preterm baby: Keep blood draws to a minimum. May be given recombinant human erythropoietin (rEPO) and supplemental iron and then iron-fortified formulas.

Symptomatic newborn: Needs increased oxygen, as do growing premature infants. Administer packed RBCs transfusion:

- Warm blood.
- Give ordered amount over greater than 30 minutes.
- Monitor for hypocalcemia and hypoglycemia.
- Do not exceed 10 mL/kg (of weight) volume per transfusion.
- Recheck hematocrit (Hct)/Hgb per agency protocol.

Polycythemia

Central venous Hct greater than 65% or Hgb greater than 20–22 g/dL and increased viscosity lead to impaired blood flow through blood vessels and decreased oxygen transport. Full-term infant with delayed cord clamping, late preterm infant, IDM, SGA, infants of preeclamptic mothers, and mothers who smoke are at risk.

Characteristics

Plethoric but cyanotic when crying. Tachypnea, tachycardia, possible murmur, congestive heart failure (CHF), respiratory distress. Decreased peripheral pulses.

Hypoglycemia, lethargy, tremors, hypotonia, poor reflexes, and possible seizures secondary to decreased cerebral perfusion. Jaundice secondary to increased RBC breakdown. Microthrombi may occur in renal and cerebral artery.

Critical Nursing Management

- Monitor pulse, respirations.
- Keep urine specific gravity less than 1.015.
- Assess color at rest and when crying.
- Obtain capillary blood sample for Hct (warming the heel before obtaining the blood helps to decrease falsely high values).
- If heel stick Hct is greater than 65%, obtain central Hct (peripheral free-flowing venous hematocrit samples are usually obtained from the antecubital fossa) for confirmation of results and to verify polycythemia.
- **If Hct greater than 65% but baby is asymptomatic:** Increase fluid intake by 20–40 mL/kg/day. Recheck heel stick Hct q6h.
- **If Hct greater than 65% and baby is symptomatic:** Assist with partial exchange transfusion (remove RBCs and replace with fresh frozen plasma or 5% albumin, or Plasmanate). The goal is to lower central venous Hct to 55%–60%.
- Monitor newborn's response to the procedure: Take vital signs (VS). *Be alert for* increased pulse, respiration rate, and temperature; signs of hypoglycemia. Obtain serial Hcts after exchange as ordered.

Jaundice

Hyperbilirubinemia is an above-normal amount of bilirubin in the blood, which, when the level is high enough, produces jaundice. Jaundice can be seen as a visible yellowing of the skin, mucosa, sclera, and urine.

- **Physiologic jaundice** is the rise in the serum bilirubin (indirect) level after the first 24 hours of life and peaking by the third to fifth day. Physiologic jaundice is common in term infants and is a result of neonatal hepatic immaturity.
- **Pathologic jaundice** is marked by yellow skin discoloration *within first 24 hours of life* and an increase in the total serum bilirubin level in term infants. The bilirubin level rises faster than 0.2 mg/dL per hr and

may continue beyond 2 weeks in full-term newborns. Total serum bilirubin concentration exceeding the 95th percentile on the phototherapy nomogram (Figure 6–2). Pathologic jaundice is most commonly associated with blood type or blood group incompatibility, infection, or biliary, hepatic, or metabolic abnormalities.

Management of Jaundice

Monitor transcutaneous bilirubin (TcB) or end tidal CO_2 (ETCO) levels. Total serum bilirubin levels must be obtained for confirmation or diagnosis of hyperbilirubinemia. Phototherapy and exchange transfusions are the primary medical treatments for hyperbilirubinemia. Phototherapy can be provided through conventional banks of phototherapy lights, by a fiber-optic blanket attached to a halogen light source around the trunk of the newborn, or by a combination of both delivery methods. (See Procedures: Infant Receiving Phototherapy, pp. 330–335.)

Nursing Assessments for Jaundice

- Assess for risk factors.

Be alert for prenatal history of Rh and ABO incompatibility; maternal use of aspirin, sulfonamides, or antimicrobial drugs; Native American, Japanese, Chinese, or Korean nationality (predisposed to higher bilirubin levels); and yellow amniotic fluid, which indicates significant hemolytic disease.

- Assess color of skin, sclera, and mucous membranes.

Assessment technique: Observe in the daylight or, using white fluorescent lights, blanch skin over bony prominence to remove capillary coloration and then assess degree of yellow discoloration. Assess oral mucosa and conjunctival sac in dark-skinned infants.

Be alert for jaundice. In the first 24 hours after birth, it mandates immediate investigation. Pallor is associated with hemolytic anemia.

- Assess total serum bilirubin laboratory results.
- Monitor bilirubin levels via (TcB) reflectance photometers or lab results.

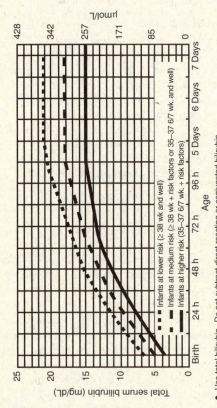

- Use total bilirubin. Do not subtract direct reacting or conjugated bilirubin.
- Risk factors = isoimmune hemolytic disease, G6PD deficiency, asphyxia, significant lethargy, temperature instability, sepsis, acidosis, or albumin < 3.0g/dL (if measured)
- For well infants 35-37 6/7 wk can adjust TSB levels for intervention around the medium risk line. It is an option to intervene at lower TSB levels for infants closer to 35 wks and at higher TSB levels for those closer to 37 6/7 wk.
- It is an option to provide conventional phototherapy in hospital or at home at TSB levels 2-3 mg/dL (35-50 mmol/L) below those shown but home phototherapy should not be used in any infant with risk factors

Infants at lower risk (≥ 38 wk and well)
Infants at medium risk (≥ 38 wk + risk factors or 35–37 6/7 wk. and well)
Infants at higher risk (35–37 6/7 wk. + risk factors)

Figure 6–2 ◼ Guidelines for phototherapy in hospitalized infants of 35 or more weeks' gestation. *Note:* These guidelines are based on limited evidence, and the levels shown are approximations. The guidelines refer to the use of intensive phototherapy, which should be used when the total serum bilirubin (TSB) exceeds the line indicated for each category. Infants are designated as "higher risk" because of the potential negative effects of the conditions listed on albumin binding of bilirubin, the blood-brain barrier, and the susceptibility of the brain cells to damage by bilirubin.

Source: From American Academy of Pediatrics Subcommittee on Hyperbilirubinemia. (2004). "Management of Hyperbilirubinemia in the Newborn Infant 35 or More Weeks of Gestation," *Pediatrics, 114*(1), 297–316, Fig. 3, p. 304.

Be alert for serum bilirubin increase of more than 0.2 mg/hr, which indicates severe hemolysis or a pathologic process. Increased reticulocytes and decreased Hct and Hgb levels are also significant.

- Assess clinical signs and symptoms.

Be alert for poor feeding, lethargy, tremors, high-pitched cry, and absent Moro reflex; these are often the first signs of bilirubin encephalopathy (kernicterus). Vomiting, irritability, rigid musculature, opisthotonos, and seizures are later signs of encephalopathy and may indicate permanent damage.

Sample Nursing Diagnoses

- *Deficient fluid volume* related to decreased intake, loose stools, and increased insensible water loss
- *Altered parenting* related to interruption in bonding between infant and parents secondary to separation

Nursing Interventions for Jaundice

Initiate feedings as soon as possible and continue q2–4h. While under phototherapy:

- Place infant under phototherapy lights unclothed, except perhaps for covering of genitals, to maximize exposure to lights. Phototherapy reduces bilirubin in the skin.

- Cover infant's eyes when under the lights. Remove eye covers once a shift with phototherapy lights off. Inspect eyes for pressure areas and conjunctivitis. Patches are removed to allow eye contact and facilitate parent–newborn interaction. Change eye patches every 24 hours. Mark patches with time, date, and right and left eye designation (to avoid cross contamination). Inspect eyes and check under the eye dressings for pressure areas.

Be alert for high-density light, which may cause retinal injury and corneal burns. Irritation from patches may cause corneal abrasions and conjunctivitis.

- Monitor VS q4h. If hypothermia or hyperthermia occurs, check temperature every hour.
- Monitor I&O q8h. Weigh infant daily (provides accurate determination of fluid intake and insensible water loss caused by phototherapy). Determine urine specific gravities q8h. Notify physician if specific gravity greater than 1.015, an indication of dehydration.

Be alert for urine specific gravity results influenced by sugar, protein, blood, and urobilinogen in the urine. Urine may be green because of the photodegradation of bilirubin. Stools are usually loose and green in color.

- Provide fluid intake 25% above normal requirements to meet increase in insensible water losses and losses in the stools. Offer D5W orally between breast-feeding or formula intake.
- Reposition infant at least every 2 hours. Monitor skin for excoriations, rash, or bronzing of the skin. Change diaper and clean area as soon after stooling as possible to prevent skin breakdown.

  Tip: Ongoing assessment of skin must be done with the phototherapy lights off.

- Turn phototherapy lights off when parents visit and for feedings. Coordinate care activities with parent visits so that parents have maximum contact with their baby with the phototherapy lights off.
- Monitor phototherapy lights' wavelength using bilimeter every shift and the number of hours each lamp is used.

- Monitor bilirubin levels per agency protocol after discontinuation of phototherapy. Turn lights off when doing bilirubin laboratory tests. Bilirubin levels may rebound following phototherapy. With the fiber-optic blanket, the light stays on at all times and the newborn is accessible for care, feeding, and diaper changes. The eyes are not covered. Fluid and weight loss are not complications of this system. Furthermore, the infant is accessible to the parents, and the therapy is less alarming to parents than standard phototherapy. A combination of a fiber-optic light source under the baby and a standard light source above has been recommended.

Evaluation

- The risks for development of hyperbilirubinemia are identified, and action is taken to minimize the potential impact of hyperbilirubinemia.
- The baby will not have any corneal irritation or drainage, skin breakdown, or major fluctuations in temperature.
- Parents will understand the rationale for, goal of, and expected outcome of therapy. Parents will verbalize their concerns about their baby's condition and identify how they can facilitate their baby's improvement.

Home Care

- Continuing care of the family with a baby experiencing jaundice is important. The nurse will assess the family's status and information needs.
- Assessments of the baby will include color, temperature, fluid status, intake, number of voidings per day, and a pattern of bowel elimination.
- Behavioral assessment is important because the baby has spent time under phototherapy, which may have interfered with normal newborn–parent interaction.
- If phototherapy lights are being used, parents must agree that the baby will be exposed to the lights for long periods of time; that they will hold the baby for only short periods for feedings, comforting, and cleansing of the perineal area; and that the room temperature will be regulated to

minimize heat loss. The nurse can assist the parents in identifying and maximizing time for interaction.

- Fiber-optic phototherapy blankets eliminate the need for eye patches, decrease heat loss because the baby is clothed, and provide more opportunities for interaction between the baby and parents. The best method of home phototherapy depends on the cause of the hyperbilirubinemia and the rate of progression of the jaundice. The nurse can assist the parents in identifying and maximizing time for interaction. Families need to be reassured that jaundice is a transient process.

NURSING CARE NEEDS OF INFANTS OF SUBSTANCE-ABUSING MOTHERS
Fetal Alcohol Syndrome (FAS)

Physical Characteristics	Early Neonatal Nursing Interventions
SGA *Abnormal features:* microcephaly, craniofacial abnormalities, postnatal growth defects, congenital heart defects, lower IQ *Withdrawal symptoms:* hyperactivity, jitteriness, lethargy, abnormal reflexes, exaggerated mouthing behaviors, inconsolable crying, abdominal distention. Delay in oral feeding development. Can start after birth and persist throughout first month of life or longer	Monitor vital signs. *Be alert for* apnea, cyanosis, and hypothermia. Provide heat conservation measures (e.g., cap for head, double wrap); for additional management, see Cold Stress discussion earlier in this chapter. Note feeding problems/patterns (offer small, frequent feedings, provide extra time). Measure abdominal girth. Be alert for abdominal distention. Place baby in dimly lit environment to prevent overstimulation. Observe for seizure activity.

SGA, small for gestational age.

Infant of a Substance-Abusing Mother (ISAM)

Physical Characteristics

SGA or premature
Withdrawal symptoms: nasal stuffiness, sneezing, yawning, increased sucking efforts

Increased secretions, difficulty feeding, drooling, gagging, vomiting, diarrhea

Increased respiratory rate, incessant cry, respiratory distress

Irritability, tremors, hyperactivity, hypertonia, hyperreflexia, increased Moro reflex, disturbed sleeping pattern

Seizures (infrequent, but may occur in severe cases or with intrauterine asphyxia)

Fever, flushing, diaphoresis

Dehydration

Early Neonatal Nursing Interventions

Assess ability to feed (hyperactivity and increased secretions cause difficulty). *Be alert for* difficult feeder with poor suck and regurgitation/vomiting.

Provide small, frequent feedings. Position on side or semi-Fowler's to prevent choking.

Note frequency of diarrhea and vomiting and weigh q8h during withdrawal.

Initiate safety precautions to prevent self-injury during periods of hyperactivity.

Observe for seizures.

Decrease stimulating activities and provide quiet environment during withdrawal period. Provide gentle handling, pacifier for non-nutritive sucking, talk in soothing voice, play quiet music, swaddle snugly with hands near mouth, and hold as much as baby tolerates.

Encourage parent-infant attachment by explaining baby's behavior and giving comfort suggestions.

Administer drugs—phenobarbital, oral morphine, oral methadone, diazepam—as ordered for relief of withdrawal symptoms. There are regional variations in medications used.

SGA, small for gestational age.

CONGENITAL HEART DEFECTS IN THE NEWBORN PERIOD

Congenital heart defects (CHDs) occur in about 1 per 1,000 live births. The CHDs seen most often in the first week of life are transposition of the great vessels and hypoplastic left heart syndrome. Within the first month of life, the presenting conditions are coarctation of the aorta, ventricular septal defect, tetralogy of Fallot, and patent ductus arteriosus. Initial assessment of the newborn suspected of having CHD includes complete physical exam, blood pressure in all four extremities, electrocardiogram (ECG), chest X-ray, and evaluation of oxygenation in 100% oxygen. Many newborns with congenital heart disease currently are diagnosed by fetal echocardiography, and corrective management can be done during the first month of life.

Management of Congenital Heart Defects

Cardiac defects of the early newborn period include the following:

Increased Pulmonary Blood Flow
Patent Ductus Arteriosus

↑ in females, maternal rubella, RDS, less than 1,500-g preterm newborns, high-altitude births

Clinical Findings	Medical/Surgical Management
Harsh grade 2–3 machinery murmur at upper left sternal border (LSB) just beneath clavicle	Indomethacin—0.2 mg/kg IV, 3 doses; one q12h (prostaglandin inhibitor)
↑ difference between systolic and diastolic pulse pressure	Surgical ligation or occlusive coils
	Use of O_2 therapy and blood transfusion to improve tissue oxygenation and perfusion

Clinical Findings	**Medical/Surgical Management**
Can lead to right heart failure and pulmonary congestion ↑ left atrial (LA) and left ventricular (LV) enlargement, dilated ascending aorta ↑ pulmonary vascularity	Fluid restriction and diuretics

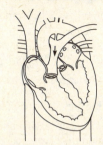

Patent Ductus Arteriosus

Obstruction to Systemic Blood Flow
Coarctation of Aorta

Can be preductal or postductal

Clinical Findings	**Medical/Surgical Management**
Absent or diminished femoral pulses Increased brachial pulses Late systolic murmur in left intrascapular area Systolic BP in lower extremities Enlarged left ventricle Can present in CHF at 7–21 days of life	Surgical resection of narrowed portion of aorta Prostaglandin E_1 to maintain peripheral perfusion No afterload reducer drugs

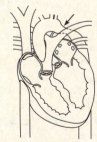

Coarctation of the Aorta

BP, blood pressure; CHF, congestive heart failure.

Decreased Pulmonary Blood Flow
Tetralogy of Fallot

(Most common cyanotic heart defect)
Pulmonary stenosis
Ventricular septal defect
Overriding aorta
Right ventricular hypertrophy

Clinical Findings	Medical/Surgical Management
May be cyanotic at birth or within first few months of life	Prevention of dehydration, intercurrent infections
Harsh systolic murmur LSB	Alleviation of paroxysmal dyspneic attacks
Crying or feeding increases cyanosis and respiratory distress	Palliative surgery to increase blood flow to the lungs
	Corrective surgery—resection of pulmonic stenosis, closure of VSD with Dacron patch
X-ray: boot-shaped appearance secondary to small pulmonary artery Right ventricular enlargement	

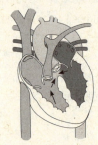

Tetralogy of Fallot

LSB, left sternal border; VSD, ventricular septal defect.

Mixed Defects
Transposition of Great Vessels (TGA)

(↑ females, IDM, low gestational ages [LGAs])

Clinical Findings	Medical/Surgical Management
Cyanosis at birth or within 3 days	Prostaglandin E_1 to vasodilate ductus to keep it open
Possible pulmonic stenosis murmur	Inotropic support
Right ventricular hypertrophy	Initial surgery to create opening between right and left side of heart if none exists
Polycythemia	Total surgical repair—usually the arterial switch done within first few days of life
"Egg on its side" X-ray	

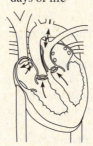

Transposition of Great Vessels

Hypoplastic Left Heart Syndrome

Clinical Findings	Medical/Surgical Management
Normal at birth—cyanosis and shock like congestive heart failure develop within a few hours to days	Palliative use of prostaglandin E_1
Soft systolic murmur just left of the sternum	Norwood procedure
Diminished pulses	Transplant
Aortic and/or mitral atresia	
Tiny, thick-walled left ventricle	
Large, dilated, hypertrophied right ventricle	
X-ray: cardiac enlargement and pulmonary venous congestion	

Nursing Assessments
for Congenital Heart Defects

Nursing assessment of the following signs and symptoms assists in identifying the newborn with a cardiac problem:

- Tachycardia: pulse over 160, may be as high as 200
- Tachypnea: reflects increased pulmonary blood flow
- Dyspnea: caused by increased pulmonary venous pressure and blood flow; can also cause chest retractions, wheezing
- Color: ashen, gray, or cyanotic
- Difficulty in feeding; requires many rest periods before finishing even 1 or 2 oz
- Failure to gain weight
- Diaphoresis: beads of perspiration over the upper lip and forehead; may accompany feeding fatigue
- Heart murmur: may not be heard in left-to-right shunting defects because the pulmonary pressure in the newborn is greater than pressure in the left side of the heart in the early newborn period
- Hepatomegaly: in right-sided heart failure, caused by venous congestion in the liver
- Cardiac enlargement

Nursing Interventions
for Congenital Heart Defects

- Give small, frequent feedings (oral) or gastric tube feeding to conserve energy (see Procedures: Performing Gavage Feeding, pp. 343–346).
- Obtain daily weights and strict I&O.

Be alert for failure to gain weight, inability to take more than an ounce of formula in 30–45 minutes of feeding, and decrease in urine output. Also note weight gain reflected as body edema.

- Provide oxygen to relieve respiratory distress. Oxygen will not remove cyanosis.

- Administer digoxin per order. Dosage should be double-checked by a second RN. It is given only after listening to the apical pulse for 1 minute and if no irregularities or slowing are noted.

  Tip: In most agencies, if infant's pulse is lower than 120 beats per minute, check with physician before giving medication.

- Diuretics (such as furosemide) are administered; potassium levels should be monitored because diuretics cause excretion of potassium.

- Morphine sulfate, 0.05 mg/kg of body weight per dose, may be given for irritability. It decreases peripheral and pulmonary resistance and therefore decreases tachypnea. Place in semi-Fowler's or knee–chest position to ease breathing.

- Fentanyl provides good pain control without the respiratory depression seen with morphine sulfate.

- Counsel parents on home care: administration of drugs, indications of drug toxicity, and measures used to prevent fatigue and promote nutrition for growth and development.

Evaluation

- Newborn's oxygen consumption and energy expenditure are minimal while at rest and during feedings.
- Newborn is protected from additional stresses such as infection, cold stress, and dehydration.
- Parents verbalize their concerns about their baby's health maintenance and need for ongoing follow-up care.

CONGENITAL ANOMALIES: IDENTIFICATION AND CARE IN NEWBORN PERIOD
Congenital Hydrocephalus (Enlarged head)

Nursing Assessments	Nursing Interventions
Enlarged or full fontanelles Split or widened sutures "Setting sun" eyes Head circumference greater than 90% on growth chart	Assess presence of hydrocephalus: measure and plot occipital-frontal baseline measurements, then measure head circumference once a day. Check fontanelle for bulging and sutures for widening. Assist with head ultrasound and transillumination. Maintain skin integrity: change position frequently. Use sheepskin pillow under head. Watch for signs of infection.

Choanal Atresia
(Occlusion of posterior nares)

Nursing Assessments	Nursing Interventions
Cyanosis and retractions at rest Snorting respirations Difficulty breathing during feeding Obstruction by thick mucus	Assess patency of nares: listen for breath sounds while holding baby's mouth closed and alternately compressing each nostril. Assist with passing feeding tube to confirm diagnosis. Maintain respiratory function: assist with taping airway in mouth to prevent respiratory distress. Position with head elevated to improve air exchange.

Cleft Lip
(Unilateral or bilateral visible defect)

Nursing Assessments

May involve external nares, nasal cartilage, nasal septum, and alveolar process
Flattening or depression of midfacial contour

Nursing Interventions

Provide nutrition: feed with special nipple.
Burp frequently (increased tendency to swallow air and reflex vomiting).
Clean cleft with sterile water (to prevent crusting on cleft prior to repair).
Support parental coping: assist parents with grief over loss of idealized baby.
Encourage verbalization of their feelings about visible defect.
Provide role model in interacting with infant. (Parents internalize others' responses to their newborn.)

Cleft Palate
(Fissure connecting oral and nasal cavity)

Nursing Assessments

May involve uvula and soft palate and extend forward to nostril, involving hard palate and maxillary alveolar ridge

Nursing Interventions

Prevent aspiration/infection: place prone or in side-lying position to facilitate drainage.
Suction nasopharyngeal cavity (to prevent aspiration or airway obstruction).

Nursing Assessments	Nursing Interventions
	During neonatal period, feed in upright position with head and chest tilted slightly backward (to aid swallowing and discourage aspiration). Provide nutrition: feed with special nipple. Burp after each ounce (tend to swallow large amounts of air).
Difficulty in sucking Expulsion of formula through nose	Clean mouth with water after feedings. Provide parental support: refer parents to community agencies and support groups. Encourage verbalization of frustrations as feeding process is long and frustrating. Praise all parental efforts. Encourage parents to seek prompt treatment for upper respiratory infection (URI) and teach them ways to decrease incidence of URI.

Tracheoesophageal Fistula (Type 3)
(Connection between trachea and esophagus)

Nursing Assessments	Nursing Goals and Interventions
History of maternal hydramnios Excessive oral secretions	Maintain respiratory status. Prevent aspiration. Quickly assess patency before putting to breast in birth area.

Nursing Assessments	Nursing Goals and Interventions
Constant drooling	Withhold feeding until esophageal patency is determined.
Abdominal distention beginning soon after birth	
Periodic choking and cyanotic episodes	Place on low intermittent suction to control saliva and mucus (to prevent aspiration pneumonia).
Immediate regurgitation of feeding	Place in warmed, humidified incubator (liquefies secretions, facilitating removal).
Clinical symptoms of aspiration pneumonia (tachypnea, retractions, rhonchi, decreased breath sounds, cyanotic spells)	Elevate head of bed 20–40 degrees (to prevent reflux of gastric juices).
Inability to pass nasogastric tube (see Figure 6–3)	Keep quiet (crying causes air to pass through fistula and to distend intestines, causing respiratory distress).
	Maintain fluid and electrolyte balance: give fluids to replace esophageal drainage and maintain hydration.
	Provide parent education. Explain staged repair: provision of gastrostomy and ligation of fistula, then repair of atresia.
	Keep parents informed; clarify and reinforce physician's explanations regarding malformation, surgical repair, pre- and postoperative care, and prognosis.
	Involve parents in care of infant and in planning for future; facilitate touch and eye contact (to dispel feelings of inadequacy, increase self-esteem and self-worth, and promote incorporation of infant into family).

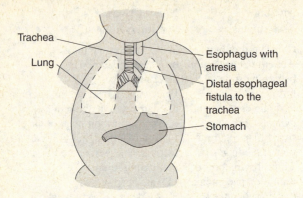

Figure 6–3 ■ The most frequently seen type of congenital tracheoesophageal fistula and esophageal atresia.

Diaphragmatic Hernia

Nursing Assessments

Difficulty initiating respirations

Gasping respirations with nasal flaring and chest retraction

Barrel chest and scaphoid abdomen

Asymmetric chest expansion

Breath sounds may be absent, usually on left side

Heart sounds displaced to right

Spasmodic attacks of cyanosis and difficulty in feeding

Nursing Interventions

Maintain respiratory status: immediately administer oxygen (O_2), may need to be intubated and ventilated.

Never ventilate with a mask and bag and O_2 because stomach and intestines will become distended with air, compressing the lungs.

Initiate gastric decompression. Assess for increased secretions around suction tube (denotes possible obstruction).

Place in high semi-Fowler's position (to use gravity to keep pressure of abdominal organs off diaphragm).

Nursing Assessments	Nursing Interventions
Bowel sounds may be heard in thoracic cavity	Turn to affected side to allow unaffected lung expansion. Carry out interventions to alleviate respiratory and metabolic acidosis.

Omphalocele (Herniation of abdominal contents into base of umbilical cord)

Nursing Assessments	Nursing Interventions
May have an enclosed transparent sac covering	Maintain hydration and temperature: provide IV D_5LR and albumin for hypovolemia. Place infant in sterile bag up to and covering defect. Initiate gastric decompression by insertion of nasogastric tube attached to low suction (to prevent distention of lower bowel and impairment of blood flow). Prevent infection and trauma to defect. Position to prevent trauma to defect. Administer broad-spectrum antibiotics.

IV, intravenous.

Myelomeningocele (Saclike cyst containing meninges, spinal cord, and nerve roots in thoracic and/or lumbar area)

Nursing Assessments	Nursing Interventions
Myelomeningocele directly connects to subarachnoid space so hydrocephalus often occurs.	Prevent trauma and infection. Position on abdomen or on side and restrain (to prevent pressure and trauma to sac).

Nursing Assessments

No response or varying response to sensation below level of sac.
May have constant dribbling of urine.
May have incontinence or retention of stool.
Anal wink may or may not be present.
Assess anterior fontanelle for bulging and fullness.

Nursing Interventions

Meticulously clean buttocks and genitals after each voiding and defecation (to decrease possibility of infection).
May put protective covering over sac (to prevent rupture and drying).
Observe sac for oozing of fluid or pus.
Observe for complications.
Credé bladder (apply downward pressure on bladder with thumbs, moving urine toward the urethra) as ordered to prevent urinary stasis.
Assess amount of sensation and movement below defect.
Obtain occipital-frontal circumference baseline measurements once a day (to detect hydrocephalus).

Developmental Dysplasia of the Hip
(Congenital dislocated hip)

Nursing Assessments

Asymmetric gluteal and anterior thigh fold
One leg may be shorter
Positive Ortolani test

Nursing Interventions

Maintain abduction position via Pavlik harness or plastic abduction splint.
Provide perineal care to prevent skin breakdown.
Instruct parents on home care.

Clubfoot

Nursing Assessments

Abnormal turning of foot/feet either inward or outward
Unable to rotate to normal position

Nursing Interventions

If casted, keep casts dry and protect legs from irritation.
Carry out circulatory and neurologic checks.
Soothe infant during and after castings.
Provide parents with cast-care instructions (handling, cleaning, and signs of complications).

Imperforate Anus

Nursing Assessments

Visible anal membrane
Inability to take rectal temperature
No passage of meconium
Abdominal distention

Nursing Interventions

Monitor for passage of first stool.
Measure abdominal girth (increasing abdominal distention).
Prepare parents for possible need for temporary colostomy.

PERINATALLY ACQUIRED NEWBORN INFECTIONS

Group B *Streptococcus*

1%–2% colonized, with 0.5% developing disease
Early onset—usually within hours of birth or within first week
Late onset—1 week to 3 months

Nursing Assessments	Nursing Interventions
Assess for severe respiratory distress (grunting and cyanosis). May become apneic or demonstrate symptoms of shock. Meconium-stained amniotic fluid seen at birth.	Closely monitor VS for signs of respiratory distress and infection. Assist with X-ray—shows aspiration pneumonia or RDS. Immediately obtain blood, gastric aspirate, external ear canal, and nasopharynx cultures. Administer antibiotics, usually aqueous penicillin or ampicillin combined with gentamicin, as soon as cultures are obtained. Early assessment and intervention are essential to survival.

Gonorrhea

Approximately 30%–35% of newborns born vaginally to infected mothers are infected. Onset 7–14 days after birth.

Nursing Assessments	Nursing Interventions
Assess for ophthalmia neonatorum (conjunctivitis). Assess for purulent discharge and corneal ulcerations. Assess for neonatal sepsis with temperature instability, poor feeding response, and/or hypotonia, jaundice.	Administer ophthalmic antibiotic ointment (see Drug Guide: Erythromycin Ophthalmic Ointment, pp. 292–293) or tetracycline. If positive maternal test, single-dose systemic antibiotic therapy (AAP & ACOG, 2007). Maintain standard precautions during procedures, educate parents regarding need for careful hand-washing. Initiate follow-up referral to evaluate any loss of vision.

IM, intramuscularly.
VS, vital signs; RDS, respiratory distress syndrome.

Chlamydia Trachomatis

Acquired during passage through birth canal.

Nursing Assessments	Nursing Interventions
Assess for perinatal history of preterm birth. Symptomatic newborns present with pneumonia—conjunctivitis (purulent yellow discharge and eyelid swelling) 5 to 14 days after birth. Assess for chronic follicular conjunctivitis (corneal neovascularization and conjunctival scarring).	Instill ophthalmic erythromycin (see Drug Guide: Erythromycin Ophthalmic Ointment, pp. 292–293). Treat chylamydial conjunctivitis or pneumonia with oral erythromycin for 14 days. Monitor for hypertropic pyloric stenosis Initiate follow-up referral for eye complications and late development of pneumonia at 4–11 weeks postnatally.

Herpes Type 2

1 in 7,500 births
Usually transmitted during vaginal birth; a few cases of in utero transmission.

Nursing Assessments	Nursing Interventions
Check perinatal history for active herpes genital lesions. Assess for small cluster of vesicular skin lesions over all the body at about 6 to 9 days of life. Disseminated form—DIC, pneumonia, hepatitis with jaundice, hepatosplenomegaly,	Carry out careful hand-washing and gown and glove isolation with linen precautions. Obtain throat, conjunctiva, cerebrospinal fluid (CSF), blood, urine, and lesion cultures to identify herpesvirus type 2 antibodies in serum IgM fraction. Cultures positive in 24–48 hours. Administer IV acyclovir (Zovirax).

Nursing Assessments	Nursing Interventions
and neurologic abnormalities. Without skin lesions, assess for fever or subnormal temperature, respiratory congestion, tachypnea, and tachycardia.	Initiate follow-up referral to evaluate potential sequelae of microcephaly, spasticity, seizures, deafness, or blindness. Encourage parental rooming-in and touching of their newborn. Show parents appropriate hand-washing procedures and precautions to be used at home if mother's lesions are active.

DIC, disseminated intravascular coagulation; IV, intravenously.

HIV/AIDS (Transplacental transmission)

Nursing Assessments	Nursing Interventions
Assess mother for risk factors: HIV-positive, infected sexual partners, drug use, or needle sharing. Assess for S & S of opportunistic infections, failure to thrive, weight loss, diarrhea, feeding intolerance, oral and genital candidiasis infection, hepatosplenomegaly, respiratory infections, lethargy, temperature instability, skin rash, lymphadenopathy, and loss of developmental milestones.	Take vital signs q4h. Maintain standard precautions per agency protocol. Avoid giving infant any injections, drawing blood, or instilling eye medication until initial bath with mild soap and water. Wear disposable gloves. Monitor stools for amount, type, consistency, change in patterns, occult blood, and reducing substances. Provide meticulous skin care and change diaper after each voiding and stooling.

Nursing Assessments	**Nursing Interventions**
Assess skin for break-down or rashes.	Provide small, frequent feedings and food supplementation.
Assess cause of parental fear.	Instruct woman and family on newborn health needs and need for routine immu-nization, except live polio vaccine.
	Determine parental under-standing of AIDS/HIV exposure.
	Provide emotional support to mother and family if breast-feeding was desired.
	Provide list of contact persons for available com-munity resources and infor-mation about current and experimental treatments.

AIDS, acquired immune deficiency syndrome; HIV, human immunodefi-ciency virus; S & S, signs and symptoms.

Oral *Candida* Infection (Thrush)

Acquired during passage through birth canal.

Nursing Assessments	**Nursing Interventions**
Assess buccal mucosa, tongue, gums, and in-side the cheeks for white plaques (at 5–7 days of age).	Differentiate white plaque areas from milk curds by using cotton-tip applicator (if it is thrush, removal of white areas causes raw bleeding areas).
Check diaper area for bright-red, well-demarcated eruptions.	Maintain cleanliness of hands, linen, clothing, diapers, and feeding apparatus.

Nursing Assessments	Nursing Interventions
Assess for thrush periodically when newborn is on long-term antibiotic therapy.	Instruct breast-feeding mothers on treating their nipples with nystatin. Administer nystatin swabbed on oral lesions 1 hr after feeding or nystatin in baby's oral cavity and on mucosa. Avoid placing gentian violet on normal mucosa; it causes irritation. Discuss with parents that gentian violet stains mouth and clothing.

REFERENCES

American Academy of Pediatrics (AAP), Committee on Fetus and Newborn & American College of Obstetricians and Gynecologists (ACOG) Committee on Obstetrics. (2007). *Guidelines for perinatal care* (6th ed.). Evanston, IL: Author.

7 THE POSTPARTAL CLIENT

The period of time (approximately 6 weeks) following childbirth, during which the body returns to a prepregnant state, is called the puerperium. Because of current practice, most women are discharged within 1–2 days after childbirth. Nursing care during this time focuses on assessment for developing complications and on client teaching. The nurse should use every opportunity to explain the normal physiologic changes to the woman so that she will be able to recognize deviations and contact her caregiver if complications arise.

POSTPARTUM NURSING ASSESSMENTS

Table 7–1 identifies the basic assessments the postpartum nurse should make, explains postpartum physiologic changes, and identifies basic teaching that is indicated.

NURSING INTERVENTIONS
FOR POSTPARTUM DISCOMFORT
Perineal Discomfort:
Episiotomy and Hemorrhoids

- Many agencies use "peri bottles" to squirt warm tap water over the woman's perineum following elimination. The woman should be taught to cleanse her perineum from the front to the back and use moist antiseptic towelettes or toilet paper in a blotting (patting) motion.
- During the first few hours after childbirth, the woman can use an ice glove or chemical ice bag on the perineal

(continued on pg. 225)

Table 7-1 Postpartum Assessment and Teaching

Physiologic Changes	Nursing Assessment	Client Teaching
Vital Signs		
Temperature: normal range; may increase to 100.4°F (38°C) because of exertion and mild dehydration.	Normal: 98–100.4°F (36.2–38°C). After first 24 hours, temperature greater than 100.4°F (38°C) suggests infection.	Advise woman that following discharge, if she experiences chills, malaise, and so forth, she should take her temperature and report fever to her caregiver.
Pulse: puerperal bradycardia may occur for 6–10 days postpartum because of decreased blood volume and cardiac strain and increased stroke volume.	Pulse: 50–90 beats per minute.	Explain that pulse slows normally.
	Tachycardia may result from difficult labor and birth or from hemorrhage. Assess for additional signs of hemorrhage.	Advise woman to report palpitations, rapid pulse.
Respirations: unchanged.	Respirations normally 12–24/min. If decreased, evaluate for medication effects; if marked tachypnea present, assess for signs of pneumonia or other respiratory disease.	Advise woman to report symptoms of complications, including difficulty breathing, cough, rapid respirations.
Blood pressure (BP): remains consistent with baseline BP. A slight decrease may indicate normal physiologic readjustment to decreased intrapelvic pressure.	BP elevated: consider pregnancy-induced hypertension, especially if accompanied by headache (see Chapter 2). Note proteinuria, edema epigastric pain, visual changes.	
	BP decreased: evaluate for additional signs of hemorrhage (rapid pulse, clammy skin).	Explain findings to woman.

Breasts

Immediately after birth, breasts are smooth, soft, and show changes in pigmentation and presence of striae, characteristics of pregnancy.

Anterior pituitary secretion of prolactin promotes milk production by stimulating alveolar cells of breast. Oxytocin, produced by posterior pituitary when infant suckles, promotes milk letdown reflex and flow of milk results. At this time breasts are producing colostrum, which is creamy and high in maternal antibodies. By 2–4 days after childbirth, the breast begins producing milk. Breasts tend to become full and hard due to milk production and venous congestion. This is called engorgement.

Assess fit and support provided by bra, which should hold all the breast tissue, and, for breast-feeding women, have cotton straps that do not stretch.

Nursing bras have flaps that open for breast-feeding.

Assess size and shape of breasts (one breast often larger than the other). Palpate and note whether breast is soft (initially), somewhat firm (associated with filling), firm (full of milk), or hard (engorgement). Note tenderness, palpable mass, heat, and edema (suggests mastitis). If present, assess for other signs of infection, including fever, malaise, or flulike symptoms. Assess nipples for fissures, cracks, blisters, soreness, inversion.

Discuss importance of wearing a well-fitting bra 24 hours a day until breast milk is suppressed in nonnursing mother or until breast-feeding mother stops nursing.

Discuss methods for relieving discomfort or engorgement for nonnursing and nursing mothers as indicated. (See Breast Engorgement in the Nonnursing Mother in this chapter, and Table 9–2.)

Review signs of infection.

(continued)

The Postpartal Client 219

Table 7-1 Postpartum Assessment and Teaching (continued)

Physiologic Changes	Nursing Assessment	Client Teaching
Abdomen		
Abdominal wall is stretched; appears loose and flabby for some time. Tone can improve in 2–3 months with exercise. Diastasis recti abdominis is a separation of the rectus abdominis muscle so that a portion of abdominal wall has no muscular support.	Abdomen feels soft, may have a "doughy" texture.	Discuss exercises that can be done to improve tone. (See discussion on page 233 and Figure 7–3.)
Uterus		
Involution: rapid reduction in size of the uterus and its return to a near prepregnant size following childbirth. Involution is enhanced by an uncomplicated birth, breast-feeding, and early ambulation. Immediately following expulsion of the placenta, uterus is contracted, about the size of a large grapefruit, located midway between symphysis and umbilicus. It gradually rises up to the level of the umbilicus as blood collects and forms clots	See Procedures: Assessing the Uterine Fundus Immediately after Birth, pp. 318–321, for correct technique. Fundus should be firm and in the midline. Displacement to the side may be caused by a full bladder. A fundus that is not firm is called "boggy." This may be caused by pressure from a full bladder, by the presence of clots, or because of diminished contractility in a woman who has borne several children. Massage fundus gently with the fingertips	Teach mother to evaluate her fundus herself. If it is boggy, she can then massage it until it is firm and report this to the nurse. Explain the importance of voiding regularly to avoid pressure on the uterus.

within the uterus. It stays there for about 1 day, then decreases in size about one finger-breadth/day. Within 10 days to 2 weeks, it is again a pelvic organ.

Muscles stay contracted to clamp off blood vessels at placental site to prevent hemorrhage.

Uterine ligaments are still stretched so uterus is movable and can be displaced by a full bladder.

Placental site takes up to 6 weeks to heal. Healing occurs by exfoliation so that no scar is formed, which would limit area available for future placental implantation.

until firm; if the uterus does not contract, more vigorous massage may be necessary; support the lower portion of the uterus above the symphysis pubis; assess bladder for distention and have woman void if necessary.

Attempt to express clots only when the uterus is firm; do not attempt to express clots from a boggy uterus. This could cause uterine inversion. If bogginess remains or returns, notify physician or nurse-midwife. Note height of uterus in relation to umbilicus and chart. Example: Uterus firm, in the midline 1 FB↑U.

(continued)

Table 7-1 Postpartum Assessment and Teaching *(continued)*

Physiologic Changes	Nursing Assessment	Client Teaching
Lochia		
After birth the uterus rids itself of the debris that remains by discharging lochia. **Lochia rubra**, which lasts for 2–3 days, is dark red, like menstrual flow. **Lochia serosa** lasts from about the 3rd to 10th day. It is similar to serosanguineous drainage. **Lochia alba**, the final discharge, is a creamy brownish or yellowish discharge.	Assess lochia for character, amount, odor (should have a slightly musty but not offensive odor; foul odor suggests infection), and the presence of clots. A few small clots are normal, but large clots are abnormal and should be investigated. Flow should never exceed moderate amount (e.g., 4–8 perineal pads daily).	Instruct woman not to use tampons postpartum because of risk of infection. Perineal pads are generally used. Explain the progression of lochia from rubra to serosa to alba. Instruct the woman to save and report excessive clots and heavily saturated pads. She should also report failure of lochia to progress from rubra to serosa or a return to rubra from serosa.
When lochia stops, the cervix is considered closed and risk of ascending infection is decreased. Lochia tends to be more abundant on arising (probably because of pooling in the vagina during the night). The amount may also increase with breast-feeding (oxytocin, released with suckling, stimulates uterine contraction) and with exertion. The type, amount, and consistency of lochia indicate the degree of healing of the placental site. Persistent	If woman reports heavy bleeding, have woman apply clean pad and reassess in 1 hour. Blood loss greater than 2 pads per hour should be reported to the CNM/physician. If she reports passage of clots, ask her to save all pads with clots and not flush toilet if clots are expelled with urination. If accurate assessment of blood loss is necessary, weigh pads after first balancing scale with a clean, dry pad; 1 g is considered equivalent to 1 mL blood.	Teach woman to change pads with each voiding or bowel movement and after showering or use of a sitz bath.

lochia rubra or a return to rubra from serosa may indicate retained placenta fragments, subinvolution, or late postpartal hemorrhage.

Perineum

Following birth, the soft tissue of the perineum may be edematous and bruised. Episiotomy may be present. Woman may also have some hemorrhoids as a result of pushing during labor.

Chart amount, followed by character. Example: Lochia: small amount, rubra, no clots.

Perineum should appear intact; slight edema and bruising are normal. Marked fullness, bruising, and pain may indicate hematoma and require further evaluation.

Inspect episiotomy laceration. There should be no redness, edema, ecchymosis, or drainage, and the edges should be well approximated.

If hemorrhoids are present, they should be small and nontender; full, reddened, inflamed hemorrhoids are painful and require comfort measures (see Perineal Discomfort: Episiotomy and Hemorrhoids in this chapter).

The woman may apply an ice glove or pack initially to prevent edema. Teach woman to use a perineal bottle filled with warm water or a surgigator after each voiding to wash the perineum and promote healing. Teach importance of wiping from the front (urinary meatus) to the back (anal area) to prevent contamination of the episiotomy laceration from the anal area. Teach comfort measures for hemorrhoids.

(continued)

Table 7–1 Postpartum Assessment and Teaching (*continued*)

Physiologic Changes	Nursing Assessment	Client Teaching
Urinary Tract		
Urinary output greatly increases in the early postpartum period because of diuresis. Woman may have difficulty voiding because of decreased bladder sensation, use of anesthesia agents during birth, swelling and bruising of tissues around urethra, increased bladder capacity, and difficulty voiding while recumbent.	Assess voiding; woman should be voiding sufficient quantities (at least 250–300 mL) every 4–6 hours; ask about symptoms of urinary tract infection (UTI) (urgency, frequency, dysuria); note whether bladder is palpable; determine whether fundus is in the midline. Palpate costovertebral angle (CVA) for tenderness.	Explain the importance of adequate voiding; help woman with difficulty by providing privacy, suggesting she pour warm water over perineum, encouraging ambulation, and describing visualization techniques. Identify symptoms of UTI; explain importance of adequate fluid intake (at least 2,000 mL) daily.
Lower Extremities		
Stasis of blood in legs due to positioning, trauma to blood vessels, and use of stirrups increase risk of thrombophlebitis. Edema is common.	Inspect legs for redness and edema. Assess for Homans' sign (pain in calf when foot sharply dorsiflexed); palpate for tenderness, warmth.	Stress the importance of early ambulation to promote venous return. Encourage woman to avoid crossing legs or using knee-gatch position on bed.
Bowel Elimination		
Bowels tend to be sluggish because of lingering effects of progesterone, decreased abdominal muscle tone, and lack of blood and fluid. Women may fear bowel movement will be painful because of episiotomy or hemorrhoids.	Ask woman about bowel elimination. She should have a normal bowel movement by second or third day after birth. Stool softeners may be indicated if hemorrhoids or episiotomy increase possibility of discomfort.	Explain importance of bowel elimination. Encourage ambulation, increased fluid intake, diet high in roughage and fiber. Explain risks of constipation.

CNM, certified nurse-midwife.

area. If a glove is used, wash it first to remove powder, then wrap it in a washcloth or towel. Leave it on 20 minutes, then off for 10 minutes.

- After the first few hours the woman can take a sitz bath, usually ordered for 20 minutes tid or qid and prn. It is soothing and cleansing, and its warmth increases circulation to promote healing.
  1. Some research suggests that a cool sitz bath may be more effective than a warm sitz bath in reducing perineal edema. Offer women a choice of temperature.
  2. Procedure: Disposable sitz tubs fit over a toilet with raised lid. At home the woman can fill a bathtub with 4–6 inches of water at a comfortable (not too hot) temperature. The bathtub should be scrubbed first, and she should not bathe in the tub water because of the risk of introducing infection.
  3. Topical agents, such as Dermoplast aerosol spray or Americaine spray, may be applied by the woman following a sitz bath.
- The previously described treatments are effective for episiotomy, lacerations, and hemorrhoids. In addition, suggested nursing interventions for hemorrhoids include the following:
  1. Encourage side-lying position.
  2. Teach the woman to reinsert hemorrhoids digitally. To do this she lies on her side, places lubricant on her finger, and applies steady gentle pressure against the hemorrhoids, pushing them inside. She should hold them in place for 1–2 minutes, then withdraw her finger. The anal sphincter should then hold them in place. She should maintain the side-lying position for a period of time.
  3. Nupercainal ointment, Tucks, or witch hazel pads may be placed against the hemorrhoids and held in place by the perineal pad. They are soothing and cool.

4. Encourage actions that help prevent constipation, such as increased fluid intake, a high-fiber diet, early ambulation, and use of stool softeners as prescribed.

Afterpains

Afterpains are the result of intermittent uterine contractions and are more common in multiparas, women who had a multiple pregnancy, and women who had hydramnios. They may be intensified by breast-feeding because oxytocin is released when the baby suckles.

- Have woman lie prone with small pillow under her abdomen. This places constant pressure on the uterus, causing it to remain contracted. Tell her the pain will be intensified for a few minutes but then will subside.
- Administer analgesic as needed. For breast-feeding women, administer about 1 hour before scheduled feeding.

Postpartum Diaphoresis

- Diaphoresis results as the body works to eliminate excess fluid and waste. It frequently occurs at night, and the woman awakens drenched with perspiration.
- Protect woman from chilling by changing bedding and providing a fresh gown.
- Encourage a shower (unless cultural practices forbid it).
- Prevent thirst by offering fluids as the woman desires.

Discomfort from Immobility

- The woman may have mild to severe muscular aches from pushing during the second stage and birth.
- Encourage early ambulation. The woman may be light-headed initially because of blood loss, fatigue, or medication, so assist her the first few times. This is especially important during the first shower, when heat may add to the problem.
- Stay close, have a call light and chair readily available, and check the woman frequently.

Suppression of Lactation
in the Nonnursing Mother

- Lactation may be suppressed through mechanical inhibition, which includes the following:
  1. Have the woman wear a well-fitting, supportive bra continuously until lactation is suppressed (about 5 days). The bra is removed only for showers. A breast binder may be applied if the woman prefers or if no bra is available.
  2. Apply ice packs over axillary area of both breasts for 20 minutes qid.
  3. Avoid any stimulation of breasts by the woman, her partner, or her infant.
  4. Avoid warmth, which stimulates milk production; avoid letting shower water flow over breasts.
  5. Parboiled cabbage leaves can be refrigerated and placed on the breast to decrease milk production.

Breast Engorgement
in the Nonnursing Mother

- Interventions are the same as those for suppression.
- Administer analgesics as necessary.

Note: Breast engorgement in the nursing mother is addressed in Chapter 9.

INFANT FEEDING
Breast-Feeding

- Physiology of lactation
  1. The hormone prolactin, from the anterior pituitary, is initially responsible for milk production.
  2. Oxytocin, from the posterior pituitary, is responsible for the letdown reflex, which triggers the flow of milk.
  3. The letdown reflex is stimulated by infant suckling, but it can also be stimulated by the newborn's presence or cry, or even thinking about the infant. It may also occur during sexual orgasm because oxytocin is released.

4. The letdown reflex may be inhibited by a mother's lack of self-confidence, feelings of fear or embarrassment, anxiety, or physical discomfort.

5. Milk production is based on the law of supply and demand. Repeated inhibition of the letdown reflex or failure to empty the breasts completely and frequently may decrease milk supply.

- Breast-feeding technique
  1. Put the newborn to breast as soon as possible.
  2. Position baby so that entire body is turned toward breast. Figure 7–1 shows a variety of positions.
  3. Direct nipple straight into infant's mouth with as much of the areola included as possible so that as infant sucks, his or her jaws compress the ducts under the areola, where milk is stored (see Figure 7–2). To do this, the mother holds the breast with her thumb placed on the upper portion and the remainder of her

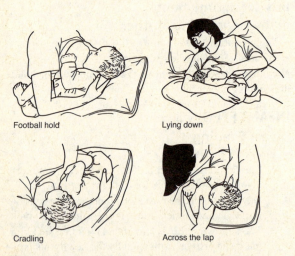

Football hold

Lying down

Cradling

Across the lap

Figure 7–1 ■ Examples of breast-feeding position changes to facilitate thorough breast emptying and to prevent nipple soreness.

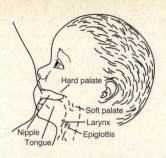

Figure 7–2 ■ To nurse effectively, it is important that the infant's mouth cover the majority of the areola to compress the ducts below. (Courtesy of Ross Laboratories, Columbus, Ohio.)

fingers cupping the breast. She then lightly strokes the infant's lips with the nipple.

4. Avoid the temptation to use a nipple shield. This confuses the baby and makes it more difficult to learn to nurse.

5. Avoid setting artificial time limits on the amount of time the baby should nurse. It may take up to 3 minutes for the letdown reflex to occur. Instead, advise the woman to let the baby nurse at one breast as long as the baby is sucking well and positioned correctly.

6. To avoid trauma to the breasts, the mother should not let the infant sleep with the nipple in his or her mouth.

7. When the baby has emptied the first breast she or he is burped and switched to the second breast. (See following discussion on Burping the Infant.) When the baby has completed feeding, she or he is burped again.

8. The baby's suck tends to be most vigorous initially. To avoid undue trauma to the breasts, the mother should alternate the breast from which she nurses first.

9. Babies are obligatory nose breathers. To avoid having the breast block the nares, the mother should either lift the breast slightly or indent the breast tissue

that is close to the baby's nose. When indenting the breast, push the tissue *toward* the baby's nose to avoid pulling the nipple out of the newborn's mouth.

10. To prevent trauma to the nipple, the mother should break suction before removing the infant from the breast by inserting a finger into the infant's mouth, next to the nipple.

11. When feeding is completed, the woman should express a small amount of milk onto the nipples, rub it into the nipples, and let nipples air dry, then inspect the nipples for trauma.

12. Frequent nursing helps establish a good supply of milk and prevents nipple trauma from the too-vigorous suck of a ravenous infant. Thus, during the first few days the mother should nurse frequently (every 1½–3 hours).

13. The mother can be encouraged to massage her breasts in a circular fashion or apply moist warm compresses to aid in letdown and prevent nipple trauma.

14. Table 9–2 identifies self-care measures a woman may use if she experiences common breast-feeding problems. See Chapter 9 for suggested interventions for other common problems.

Formula Feeding

- Formula feeding is also a nurturing choice for infant feeding and allows both parents to share in this nurturing activity with their child. A variety of commercial formulas are available.

- Whole milk and skim milk should not be used for children under 2 years. Whole milk has too high of a protein content; skim milk also has too much protein and lacks adequate calories and essential fatty acids.

- Formula tends to be digested more slowly, so the bottle-fed infant may go longer between feedings. Infants are usually fed "on demand," which typically is every 3–5 hours.

- Formula-feeding technique
  1. The mother should assume a comfortable position with adequate arm support so that she can cradle her baby in her arm close to her body.
  2. The bottle should be held, not propped, with the baby's head somewhat elevated. Feeding the infant horizontally may result in positional otitis media.
  3. The nipple should have a large enough hole to permit milk to flow in drops when the bottle is inverted. Too large of an opening may cause overfeeding and regurgitation.
  4. The nipple should be pointed directly into the mouth and on top of the tongue. It should be kept full of formula to avoid ingestion of extra air.
  5. The infant should be burped at regular intervals, preferably at the middle and end of the feeding, or, during the first few feedings, after about every ½ oz. If the infant was crying vigorously before feeding, he or she should be burped before feeding or after taking just enough formula to calm down. (See following discussion on Burping the Infant.)
  6. Infants should be encouraged, but not forced, to feed. Overfeeding can lead to infant obesity.
  7. Nutritive additives, such as rice or infant cereal, should not be added to the formula.

Burping the Infant

- Burping is done by holding the infant upright on the shoulder or by holding the infant in a sitting position on the feeder's lap with the chin and chest supported by one hand. The back is then stroked or patted gently.
- Newborns frequently regurgitate small amounts. The feeder may find it helpful to keep a "burp cloth" handy. Forceful emesis requires medical evaluation, especially if other symptoms are present.

THE Rh-NEGATIVE MOTHER

- A woman who is Rh negative with an indirect Coombs' test negative, and whose infant is Rh positive with a direct Coombs' test negative, is given RhIG (RhoGAM) within 72 hours after childbirth.

- See Procedures: Administration of Rh Immune Globulin (RhoGAM, HypRho-D), pp. 313–315.

RUBELLA VACCINE

- Women who are not immune to rubella (German measles), as evidenced by a titer of less than 1:10, are usually given the rubella vaccine during the immediate postpartal period because it is known that they are not pregnant.
- Because the rubella vaccine is a live, attenuated vaccine, women are advised not to become pregnant for at least 3–4 months after receiving it.

POSTPARTAL EXERCISES

- The woman should be encouraged to begin simple exercises in the hospital and to continue them at home. Exercise helps to improve muscle tone, contributes to postpartum weight loss, and aids in preventing constipation. Many agencies have a booklet on appropriate exercises.

Figure 7–3 identifies some commonly used exercises.

SIBLING PREPARATION FOR THE NEWBORN

- Sibling visits reassure the children that their mother is well and still loves them.
- The parents may ask for advice about dealing with the siblings when mother and baby return from the hospital. The following advice may be helpful:
  1. If possible, have the father carry the new baby inside so that the mother's arms are free to embrace her other children.
  2. Some mothers bring a doll home for the older sibling. The sibling can then care for the doll when the mother is caring for the baby.
  3. Involving older children in baby care helps them develop a sense of closeness with the baby. Even very young children can hold the baby with supervision.

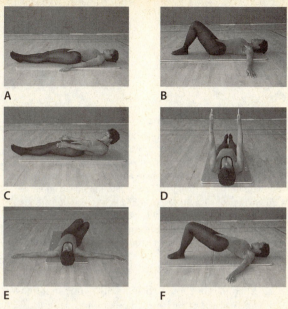

Figure 7–3 ■ Postpartal exercises. Begin with 5 repetitions two or three times daily and gradually increase to 10 repetitions. On the first day the woman should do the following: **A,** Abdominal breathing. Lying supine, inhale deeply using the abdominal muscles. The abdomen should expand. Then exhale slowly through pursed lips, tightening the abdominal muscles. **B,** Pelvic rocking. Lying supine with arms at sides, knees bent, and feet flat, tighten the abdomen and buttocks and attempt to flatten back on floor. Hold for a count of 10, then arch the back, causing the pelvis to "rock." On the second day add the following exercises: **C,** Chin to chest. Lying supine with legs straight, raise head and attempt to touch chin to chest. Slowly lower head. **D,** Arm raises. Lying supine, arms extended at 90-degree angle from body, raise arms so that they are perpendicular and hands touch. Lower slowly. On fourth day add the following: **E,** Knee rolls. Lying supine with knees bent, feet flat, and arms extended to the side, roll knees slowly to one side, keeping shoulders flat. Return to original position and then roll to opposite side. **F,** Buttocks lift. Lying supine, arms at sides, knees bent, and feet flat, slowly raise buttocks and arch the back. Return slowly to the starting position. (*continued*)

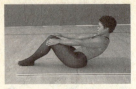
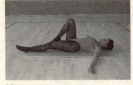

G   **H**

Figure 7–3 (continued) ■ On the sixth day add the
following: **G,** Abdominal tighteners. Lying supine, knees bent,
and feet flat, slowly raise head toward knees. Arms should extend
along either side of legs. Return slowly to original position.
H, Knee to abdomen. Lying supine, arms at sides, bend one knee
and thigh until foot touches buttocks. Straighten leg and lower
it slowly. Repeat with other leg. After 2–3 weeks, more strenuous
exercises such as sit-ups and side leg raises may be added as
tolerated. Kegel exercises, begun antepartally, should be done
many times daily during postpartum to restore vaginal and
perineal tone.

4. Each parent should spend quality time in a one-to-
   one experience with each older child. Hugs, kisses,
   and words of praise are also important.
5. Regression is common, and a toilet-trained child
   may regress or may request a bottle for meals.

RESUMPTION OF SEXUAL ACTIVITY

- Advise couple to abstain from sexual intercourse until
  the episiotomy is healed and the lochia has stopped—
  usually by the end of the third week. Many providers
  recommend refraining from intercourse until after the
  6-week check-up.
- Some form of water-soluble lubricant such as K-Y jelly
  may be necessary for intercourse to prevent discomfort
  because the vagina may be dry (hormone poor).
- Warn breast-feeding couples that the woman may leak
  milk with orgasm because of the release of oxytocin.
  Some couples find this pleasurable or amusing; others
  prefer to have the woman wear a bra. Nursing the baby
  before intercourse may help prevent leaking.

- Point out that the woman may experience decreased interest in sex due to hormonal changes, fatigue, dissatisfaction with her personal appearance, and lingering discomfort (often related to the episiotomy). This may be frustrating, especially for her partner, and the couple may find it helpful to discuss the issue openly.
- To avoid an unplanned pregnancy, advise the couple to use contraception when they resume sexual activity, even if the woman's menses has not yet returned (see Chapter 8).

CARE OF THE WOMAN FOLLOWING CESAREAN BIRTH

- The new mother who has given birth by cesarean has postpartal needs similar to those of women who give birth vaginally; however, she also has nursing care needs similar to those of women who have undergone major abdominal surgery.
- Nursing interventions include the following:
  1. Encourage the woman to cough, breathe deeply, and use incentive spirometry every 2–4 hours while awake for the first day or two following birth.
  2. Encourage leg exercises every 2 hours until the woman is ambulatory.
  3. Monitor temperature for fever (infection), blood pressure for decrease, and pulse for increase (hemorrhage).
  4. Elevated blood pressure may indicate preeclampsia (may occur for up to 48 hours postpartum).
  5. Assess for adequate voiding after the Foley catheter is removed. Implement nursing interventions if necessary to encourage voiding (privacy, increased fluid, warm water over perineum, ambulation).
  6. Assess for evidence of abdominal distention. Note presence or absence of bowel sounds. Measures to prevent or minimize gas pains include leg exercises, abdominal tightening, early ambulation, and avoiding the use of straws.

7. Flatulence may be relieved by lying on the left side, using a rocking chair, assuming a hands and knees position with the buttocks elevated, and using anti-flatulents (such as simethicone), suppositories, and enemas.

8. Encourage shower by second postpartal day. The mother can be advised to remove the dressing while showering to decrease discomfort. Stay close in case the woman becomes faint. The incision should be inspected after the dressing is removed.

9. Measures to alleviate pain include the following:

   a. Administer analgesics as needed. Patient-controlled analgesia (PCA) is frequently used. Epidural anesthesia may be used for the first 12–24 hours immediately after the cesarean. This method provides pain relief for at least 24 hours.

   b. Offer comfort through positioning, back rubs, oral care, and reduction of noxious stimuli such as noise or odors.

   c. Encourage presence of significant others, including baby.

   d. Encourage breathing, relaxation, and distraction techniques (such as those taught in childbirth preparation classes).

- Provide opportunities for parent–infant interaction.
- Discharge teaching includes need for adequate rest, warning signs of infection, and ways of lifting and feeding infant to avoid strain.

8 FAMILY PLANNING

Family planning refers to actions an individual or a couple take to avoid a pregnancy, to space future pregnancies for a specific reason, or to gain control over the number of children conceived. Thus, at a given time a woman may choose one method of contraception, and at a later time may elect to use a different approach. Family planning is often addressed during well-woman examinations; however, the information is also an important part of care during the postpartum period.

OVERVIEW

- The decision to use a method of contraception may be made individually by a woman (or, in the case of condoms or vasectomy, by a man) or jointly by a couple.
- Contraceptive information should be made available before the woman is discharged.
- In choosing a method, consistency of use outweighs absolute reliability of a given method.
- Review for the woman (or couple) the advantages and disadvantages of each method, risk factors and contraindications, and the ways of using a given method.
  Note: Different methods of contraception may be appropriate at different times in the couple's life. Table 8–1 identifies factors to consider in selecting a method of contraception.

SPERMICIDES

- Spermicides provide contraceptive protection by destroying sperm or neutralizing vaginal secretions and thereby immobilizing sperm.

Table 8–1   Factors to Consider in Choosing a Method of Contraception

Effectiveness of method in preventing pregnancy

Safety of the method

  Are there inherent risks?

  Does it offer protection against STIs or other conditions?

Client's age and future childbearing plans

Any contraindications in client's health history

Religious or moral factors influencing choice

Personal preferences or biases

Lifestyle

  How frequently does client have intercourse?

  Does she have multiple partners?

  Does she have ready access to medical care in the event of complications?

  Is cost a factor?

Partner's support and willingness to cooperate

Personal motivation to use method

STIs, sexually transmitted infections

- The spermicide available for use in the United States, nonoxynl-9 (N-9), is available in a variety of forms, including cream, foam, jelly, film, and suppositories.
- Spermicides are only minimally effective when used alone. Effectiveness increases when used with a male condom, diaphragm, cervical cap, or female condom.
- Advantages
  1. Wide availability and low toxicity
- Disadvantages
  1. Low reliability
  2. Some messiness
  3. Does not offer protection from the human immunodeficiency (HIV) virus or from any other sexually transmitted infection. N-9 may actually increase a woman's risk of HIV infection because it irritates vaginal tissue, making it more susceptible to invasion by organisms such as HIV (FDA, 2007).

BARRIER METHODS OF CONTRACEPTION

- Barrier methods prevent the transport of sperm to the ovum, immobilize sperm, or are lethal against them.
- Methods include condoms, diaphragm, cervical cap, and vaginal sponge.
- Barrier methods are often used in conjunction with spermicides, which some authorities consider a form of chemical barrier.
- Barrier methods are clearly related to an individual's sexual behavior. Each act of intercourse demands that one or both partners consciously decide whether to use a barrier contraceptive and then take action.
- Barrier methods of contraception are a good choice for women who:
  1. Have a contraindication to using a specific method such as combined oral contraceptives (COCs), intrauterine device (IUD), subdermal implants, and the like
  2. Are opposed to taking systemic medications or chemicals such as COCs, monthly injections, and so forth
  3. Are in early postpartum or are lactating
  4. Need a back-up method of contraception for a period of time, such as when beginning COCs, after an IUD has been inserted, or when a male partner has just had a vasectomy
  5. Have intercourse rarely or sporadically
  6. Are perimenopausal smokers and thus not good candidates for COCs.

Male Condom

- Effectiveness is increased when male condom is used in combination with a spermicide.
- Advantages
  1. Small, lightweight, disposable, and inexpensive
  2. No side effects
  3. Requires no medical examination or supervision
  4. Offers visual evidence of effectiveness

5. Provides some protection against sexually transmitted infections (STIs).
- Disadvantages
  1. Risk of breakage or displacement
  2. Possible perineal or vaginal irritation
  3. Some dulling of sensation
- Method of use
  1. Condoms are applied to the erect penis and rolled from the tip to the end of the shaft before vulvar or vaginal contact is made.
  2. A small space is left at the tip to accommodate ejaculate, thereby preventing breakage.
  3. Condom rim should be held when penis is withdrawn from vagina to prevent spillage.
  4. Latex may be weakened by prolonged exposure to heat.

Note: Only latex condoms offer protection against human immunodeficiency virus/acquired immune deficiency syndrome. "Skin condoms" made of lamb intestine do not.

Female Condom
- This is a barrier method; it is not designed to be used with a male condom.
- Advantages
  1. See male condom discussion.
  2. Because it covers a portion of the woman's perineum and the base of the penis during intercourse, it may offer increased protection against STIs.
- Disadvantages
  1. Higher cost, noisiness during intercourse, cumbersome feel.
- Method of use
  1. Thin polyurethane sheath with a flexible ring at each end. Inner ring serves as a means of insertion and covers the cervix like a diaphragm.
  2. Second ring remains outside vagina and covers a portion of the perineum.

3. Inner sheath prelubricated.
4. May be inserted up to 8 hours before intercourse (see Figure 8–1).

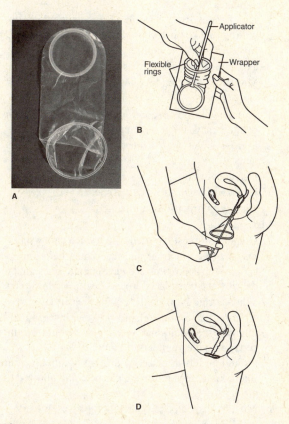

Figure 8–1 ■ **A,** The female condom. To insert the condom: **B,** Remove condom and applicator from wrapper by pulling up on the ring. **C,** Insert condom slowly by gently pushing the applicator toward the small of the back. **D,** When properly inserted, the outer ring should rest on the folds of skin around the vaginal opening, and the inner ring (closed end) should fit loosely against the cervix.

Diaphragm

- Barrier contraceptive
- Used with a spermicidal cream or jelly
- Advantages
  1. Excellent choice for women who are unable or unwilling to take birth control pills or to have an IUD
  2. Involves no medication
  3. Contraception only used as necessary
  4. May be inserted up to 4 hours before intercourse
- Disadvantages
  1. Women who are not comfortable manipulating their genitals may find it unacceptable.
  2. Some couples feel it interferes with sexual spontaneity.
- Contraindications
  1. History of toxic shock syndrome
  2. History of urinary tract infections
- Method of use
  1. Diaphragm must be fitted by a trained caregiver.
  2. Diaphragm is inserted into the vagina before intercourse with approximately 1 teaspoonful of spermicidal jelly or cream placed around the rim and in the cup.
  3. When correctly placed, it covers the cervix.
  4. If more than 6 hours elapse between insertion and intercourse, additional spermicide should be inserted into the vagina (see Figure 8–2).
  5. Should be left in place for at least 6–8 hours after intercourse, then removed, cleaned, and allowed to air dry.
  6. Must be inspected periodically for holes or tears.

Cervical Cap

- The cervical cap is similar to the diaphragm, except it fits snugly over the cervix.
- Cap may be left in place for up to 48 hours, but most caregivers recommend that it not be left in place for more than 24 hours.

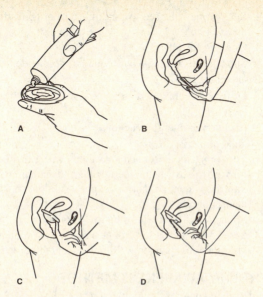

Figure 8–2 ■ Inserting the diaphragm. **A,** Apply jelly to the rim and center of the diaphragm. **B,** Insert the diaphragm. **C,** Push the rim of the diaphragm under the pubic symphysis. **D,** Check placement of the diaphragm. The cervix should be felt through the diaphragm.

- Repeated acts of intercourse do not require additional spermicide.
- Cap tends to be more difficult than the diaphragm for women to insert and remove.

Vaginal Sponge

- The vaginal sponge is a pillow-shaped, soft, absorbent synthetic sponge containing the spermicide N-9.
- It is made with a concave or cupped area on one side, which is designed to fit over the cervix. It also has a loop to permit easy removal.
- Advantages
  1. Professional fitting is not required.

2. Sponge may be used for multiple acts of coitus for up to 24 hours.
3. One size fits all.
4. Sponge acts as both a barrier and a spermicide.
- Disadvantages
   1. Difficulty removing it
   2. Cost
   3. Irritation or allergic reactions
- Method of use
   1. The sponge is moistened thoroughly with water before use to activate the spermicide, and then inserted into the vagina so that the cupped side fits snugly against the cervical os.
   2. Sponge may be worn for up to 24 hours.
   3. Sponge should be left in place for at least 6 hours after intercourse and then removed and discarded.

FERTILITY AWARENESS METHODS
- Also called natural family planning
- Include calendar method (also called rhythm), basal body temperature method, cervical mucus method, and symptothermal method
- Advantages
   1. Free, safe, and acceptable to many whose religious beliefs prohibit other methods
   2. Involves no artificial substances or medications
   3. Encourages a couple to communicate about sexual activity and family planning
   4. Useful in helping a family plan a pregnancy
- Disadvantages
   1. Requires extensive initial counseling to use effectively
   2. May interfere with sexual spontaneity
   3. Requires extensive maintenance of records for several cycles before beginning use
   4. Difficult for women with irregular cycles to use
   5. Not as reliable as other methods

- Method of use: Changes in a woman's cycle (such as changes in mucus, temperature, and so forth) are used to identify fertile and safe days.

INTRAUTERINE DEVICE

- Is a true contraceptive; IUD triggers a spermicidal-type reaction in the body, thereby preventing fertilization.
- The IUD also produces a local inflammatory effect on the endometrium.
- It is best suited for multiparous women in a monogamous relationship, although at the request of the company that manufactures the Copper T380A, the FDA removed a "patient or partner with multiple sexual partners" as a contraindication for its use. This change can apply as well to the LNG-IUS (Ogburn & Esprey, 2007).
- Research indicates that, contrary to common belief, the IUD is reliable and effective for women who have never been pregnant, it is effective against ectopic pregnancy because of its overall effectiveness in preventing any pregnancy, and the copper IUD is a good choice for women who cannot use hormonal forms of contraception (Jacobstein, 2007).
- Types available: copper-containing Cu380T (Para-Gard) and levonorgestrel-releasing intrauterine system (Mirena)
- Advantages
  1. Highly effective
  2. Continuous contraceptive protection
  3. No coitus-related activity
  4. Relatively inexpensive over time
- Disadvantages
  1. IUD increases risk of pelvic inflammatory disease (PID) in women with multiple partners.
  2. Side effects may include severe dysmenorrhea, irregular menses, increased bleeding during menses, uterine perforation, and expulsion of the IUD.

3. If IUD fails and pregnancy results, the device should be removed as soon as possible to prevent infection.
- Contraindications
  1. History of PID
  2. Not the preferred choice for women with multiple sexual partners because of the increased risk of PID
- Method of use
  1. IUD requires signed consent before insertion by a physician, certified nurse-midwife, or trained nurse practitioner.
  2. The woman should check for the presence of the string once weekly for the first month and then after each menses.

COMBINATION ESTROGEN-PROGESTIN APPROACHES

- The use of a combination of the hormones estrogen and progesterone is a highly successful, very safe birth control method.
- Hormonal contraceptives work by inhibiting the release of an ovum, by creating an atrophic endometrium, and by maintaining a thick cervical mucus that slows sperm transport and inhibits the process that allows sperm to penetrate the ovum.
- Several forms are available, including COCs, transdermal patches, vaginal rings, injections, and implants.

Combined Oral Contraceptives (Birth control pills)

- Advantages
  1. No coitus-related activity
  2. High effectiveness rate
  3. Noncontraceptive benefits include decreased menstrual cramps, decreased menstrual flow, increased cycle regularity, decreased incidence of functional ovarian cysts; also substantially reduced incidence of ectopic pregnancy, ovarian cancer, endometrial

cancer, iron deficiency anemia, and benign breast disease.

- Disadvantages
  1. Pills must be taken daily.
  2. Oral contraceptives have some serious associated side effects, especially those related to thrombus formation.
- Contraindications
  1. Pregnancy
  2. Previous history of thrombophlebitis, acute or chronic liver disease, presence of estrogen-dependent carcinoma, undiagnosed uterine bleeding, heavy smoking, hypertension, diabetes, and hyperlipidemia
- Method of use
  1. Pills are prescribed after a careful review of the woman's history and a thorough physical exam, including blood pressure check and Pap smear.
  2. Woman is seen yearly while on the pill.
  3. Pills are generally begun on the first Sunday after the beginning of the menstrual cycle and are taken daily for 21 days. The woman then stops for 1 week (or takes seven "blank" pills if she prefers a 28-day package). She then resumes taking the pills.
  4. Low-dose pills should be taken within 4 hours of the same time daily.
  5. Woman should use a back-up method such as condoms during her first cycle on the pills.
  6. If a pill is missed, woman should take it when she remembers and take her pill for the day at the regular time.
  7. Many women take their pills at night, when they are less rushed, and so they are asleep when most side effects (such as nausea) would occur.

Note: Seasonale® is a COC marketed for extended use. Women using Seasonale take 84 active pills followed by 7 blank pills. These women have 4 periods per year instead of 12.

Transdermal Hormonal Contraception

- The contraceptive skin patch is called Ortho Evra.
- The patch is applied weekly for 3 weeks on one of four sites: the woman's abdomen, buttocks, upper outer arm, or trunk (excluding the breasts).
- During the fourth week, no patch is applied and menses typically occurs.
- The patch is as safe and effective as COCs and has a better rate of user compliance.
- Women who are candidates for COCs are candidates for the patch unless they are obese (weight greater than 198 lb).

Vaginal Contraceptive Ring

- The NuvaRing vaginal contraceptive ring (manufactured by Organon Inc.) is a flexible, soft vaginal ring that is inserted monthly.
- The ring is left in place for 21 days and then removed for 7 days.
- One size fits virtually all women.

Injectible Combination Contraceptive

- Called Lunelle (medroxyprogesterone acetate and estradiol cypionate), this form of contraception is off the market in the United States because of manufacturing problems.
- The monthly intramuscular injection is highly effective.
- The side effect pattern is similar to that of COCs.

LONG-ACTING PROGESTIN CONTRACEPTIVES

- Types
  1. Subdermal implants are not currently available in the United States. Rods containing levonorgestrel are implanted in a woman's arm. Norplant, a six-rod system, Jadelle, a two-rod system, and Implanon, a single-rod system, are available in Europe.

2. Depot-medroxyprogesterone acetate (DMPA; Depo-Provera): a singular intramuscular injection is given every 3 months.
- Method of action
  1. Prevents ovulation in most women
  2. Also stimulates the production of thick cervical mucus, which inhibits sperm penetration
- Advantages
  1. Provides continuous contraception that is removed from the act of coitus
  2. Long acting
- Disadvantages
  1. Variety of side effects (spotting or irregular bleeding, amenorrhea, weight gain, increased incidence of ovarian cysts, hirsutism, headaches, depression) may occur.
  2. Implants may be visible in very slender users; may be difficult to remove.
  3. With DMPA, return of fertility may be delayed up to 5 months.
  4. DMPA is not recommended for use longer than 2 years because it has been associated with calcium loss from bones that may not resolve after discontinuing use.

EMERGENCY POSTCOITAL CONTRACEPTION

- Emergency contraception is indicated when a woman is worried about pregnancy because of unprotected intercourse, rape, or possible contraceptive failure (e.g., broken condom, slipped diaphragm, missed oral contraceptives, or too long a time between DMPA injections).
- Emergency contraception taken within 72 hours can reduce the risk of pregnancy after a single act of unprotected intercourse by 89% (Office of Population Research & Association of Reproductive Health Professionals, 2007).

- Though sometimes called the "morning-after pill," this is misleading because the woman actually takes two pills as soon after intercourse as possible and two more 12 hours later.
- Two product kits, Preven, a combined hormonal approach (levonorgestrel and ethinyl estradiol), and Plan B, a progestin-only approach (levonorgestrel), are now approved by the FDA for emergency contraception.
- Information about postcoital emergency contraception is available through the Emergency Contraception Hotline (1-888-NOT-2-LATE), and on the World Wide Web.

OPERATIVE STERILIZATION
- This inclusive term refers to surgical procedures that permanently prevent pregnancy.
- Two types exist: vasectomy (in males) and tubal ligation (in females).
- Even though each procedure is theoretically reversible, the permanency of it should be stressed and understood.

Vasectomy
- The male sterilization procedure severs the vas deferens surgically.
- This relatively simple procedure does not interfere with erectile function.

Tubal Ligation
- The female sterilization procedure severs the fallopian tubes.
- Because it involves general anesthesia, it has more associated risks than vasectomy.

REFERENCES

Food and Drug Administration (FDA). (2007). Over-the-counter vaginal contraceptive and spermicide drug products containing nonoxynol 9; required labeling. Final rule. *Federal Register, 72*(243), 71769–71785.

Jacobstein, R. (2007). Long-acting and permanent sterilization: An international development, service delivery perspective. *Journal of Midwifery & Women's Health, 52*(4), 361–367.

Office of Population Research & Association of Reproductive Health Professionals. (2007). Emergency contraception pills ("morning after pills"). Retrieved September 9, 2007, from http://ec.princeton.edu/info/ecp.html.

9   HOME CARE OF THE
POSTPARTAL FAMILY

OVERVIEW

Home care for the postpartum family is focused more on assessment, teaching, and counseling than on physical care. The home setting allows the nurse and family to interact in a more relaxed environment, one in which the family has control. The challenges of assessing and enhancing self-care and/or infant care may be quite unique in the home, and the nurse will have many opportunities to use critical thinking skills to develop creative options with the family.

PLANNING THE HOME VISIT

The nurse should:

- Plan the home visit to occur within 24–48 hours after discharge.
- Make sure the family is consulted regarding a home visit, and the time is planned with the family members.
- Explain the purpose of the visit.
- Plan the content to be addressed and gather anticipated materials and equipment.
- Think of ways to create and foster relationships with the family.
- Employ safety measures when preplanning and executing the visit.
- Be familiar with various cultural norms and traditions.

- Document the visit to include the maternal physical and psychologic status and self-care and newborn-care teaching needs met.
- Provide telephone follow-up.

MAINTAINING SAFETY DURING A HOME VISIT

Safety is a concern regardless of where nurses are interacting with clients; however, additional precautions can be taken to increase personal safety while out in the community. These precautions include the following:

- Know the specific address and ask a family member for detailed directions to the home.
- Trace the route on a map before leaving and take the map along. Take time to drive around the neighborhood before the visit to identify potential problems.
- Notify someone when you are leaving for a visit and check in with that person as soon as the visit is completed.
- Ensure that your vehicle is well maintained and has sufficient fuel.
- Carry a cellular phone or some method of communication. (Be sure the battery is charged.)
- Carry a phone card or enough change to make a call from a pay phone if needed.
- Lock valuables, including your purse, out of sight in the trunk before you arrive at the destination.
- Have a working flashlight available, especially if making evening visits.
- In accordance with agency policy, wear scrubs, a lab coat, or other uniform that identifies you as a nurse. Wear a name tag and sensible shoes. Avoid wearing expensive jewelry.
- Be aware of personal body language and be alert to the body language of anyone present during the visit, not just the new mother.

- Leave the home immediately if a gun or knife is visible and the client or family member refuses requests to put it away.
- Convey a sense of respect at all times.
- If an occasion occurs that feels unsafe, end the visit.

NURSING ASSESSMENTS IN THE HOME

The unique aspect of home care is that the nurse is practicing alone. Critical thinking and appropriate communication skills are essential.

- Observe family dynamics. Who is the primary caregiver? Who makes the decisions regarding care of the newborn? Are siblings involved? How are siblings included in interactions and care of the new baby? How is communication shared?
- What information do the parents think they need? It is important to begin with the parents' questions.
- Is the home a safe environment for the newborn and the rest of the family? Where does the baby sleep? Are referrals needed and desired?

HOME CARE OF THE NEWBORN

- Complete a newborn assessment. Determine vital signs and assess fontanelles, color, evidence of jaundice, skin condition, the umbilical cord, circumcision if done, reflexes (suck, grasp, and moro), nutritional status and feeding, elimination, activity, sleep-wake cycles, and weight.
- The family should have been taught all necessary caregiving methods before discharge, but during the home visit you may use a checklist to determine that the family clearly understands the material.
- Review methods of obtaining the newborn's temperature. Provide an opportunity for the parents to demonstrate taking the baby's temperature if they feel comfortable doing so.
- Review holding techniques and determine if the parents have questions.

- Review positioning of the newborn for comfort and safety such as "Back to Sleep Guidelines" and need for "tummy time."
- Review cord care, perineal care with diaper changes, and circumcision care (if applicable).
- Demonstrate a newborn bath if indicated.

NEWBORN BATH

- Collect supplies (see Table 9–1).
- Advise parents to schedule uninterrupted time for the bath, if possible.
- Wash baby's face using a washcloth that has been moistened in warm water but does not contain soap.
- Cleanse eyes first (while the washcloth is the most clean). Using a corner of the washcloth around your finger, wipe the right eye from the inner canthus to the outer canthus, in one stroke. If another swipe is needed, use another corner of the washcloth. The left eye is washed in the same manner.
- Wash remainder of face, as well as under the chin. Dry. The baby's hair may be washed now or at the end of the bath. (Those most interested in organization and saving steps would say to shampoo the hair now; others would say it needs to be done at the end of the bath to better maintain the newborn's temperature.)
- Wash the chest and abdomen using either lathered hands or a washcloth, then rinse and dry.
- Complete umbilical care per agency protocol. Research shows that keeping the cord clean and dry is best (AAP & ACOG, 2007).

Table 9–1   Bath Supplies

A plastic tub	Ointments containing
Two bath towels for baby	vitamins A and D
Two washcloths	(for dry skin)
Mild soap (unperfumed is best	Cotton balls or cotton
because it is not as drying to	swabs for cleansing cord
the baby's skin)	

- Remove diaper. If bathing a male baby, be sure to keep a diaper or cloth at hand in case the baby urinates (a male infant is able to spray the urine on a caregiver).
- Gently clean from the area of the symphysis (pubic bone) down toward the anus. Use a separate portion of the washcloth for each motion. The baby's back and buttocks may be washed, rinsed, and dried.

Note: Baby powder (or cornstarch) is not recommended for diaper rash. Baby powder may cake with urine and irritate the perineal area. Cornstarch may promote fungal infection.

- If the hair has not yet been washed, carefully wrap the baby in a dry blanket. Use a football hold to support the baby safely and yet have one hand free for shampooing. Wet the baby's hair and apply a mild shampoo. Lather, rinse thoroughly, and dry. Brushing the baby's hair stimulates the scalp and also removes dead skin cells and prevents cradle cap.
- Make a hood over the baby's head until he or she is completely dressed and rewarmed after the bath to help retain the infant's body temperature.
- Review procedure for cutting the nails. The nails may be trimmed with special baby-sized cuticle/nail scissors. (Clippers may be too large to allow you to see the baby's nails.)

SLEEP SAFETY

- Sudden infant death syndrome (SIDS) is the primary cause of infant death beyond the neonatal period in the United States.
- The SIDS risk factors with the greatest potential for modification include prone sleeping position, sleeping on soft surfaces, maternal smoking (especially during pregnancy), and overheating (AAP, 2005). Thus, infants should sleep in nonprone positions (supine) and on a firm mattress.
- Infants may be given a pacifier to further prevent sudden infant death syndrome.

- Soft blankets and stuffed animals should be removed from the crib.
- Infants should sleep in the parent's room or in an area close to the parents so the parents can hear if there is a breathing problem. Cosleeping is not recommended (AAP Task Force, 2005).
- The crib headboard and footboard should be solid, with no large designs cut out of the wood, as the infant's head could become entrapped in them. Crib slats should be no more than 2⅜ inches apart.
- Mattresses should fit snugly to prevent the baby from becoming entrapped and suffocating. Side rails should always be kept up.
- Review need for Newborn Screening and Immunization follow up (see Chapter 5 for information).

HOME CARE OF THE MOTHER

- Complete a physical and psychosocial assessment.
- Ask specifically about the following areas: (1) progression of lochia (color, amount of flow, presence of foul odor or clots); (2) fever or malaise; (3) dysuria or difficulty voiding; (4) pain in the pelvis or perineum; (5) painful, reddened hot spots or shooting pains in the breasts during or between feedings; (6) areas of redness, edema, tenderness, or warmth in the legs.
- Determine questions the mother has and provide information.
- Determine if the home environment is safe. Assess all postpartum women for domestic and family violence.
- Determine if the woman has any signs of postpartum depression.
- Reinforce teaching about postpartum exercises.
- Discuss infant feeding techniques and provide assistance as needed. See the Infant Feeding section in Chapter 7 for additional information.
- Determine if assistance and support for the mother are available and if additional assistance is needed.

Table 9–2 Self-Care Measures for the Woman with Breast-Feeding Problems

Nipple Inversion

Use special breast shields such as Woolrich or Eschmann.

Use hand to shape nipple when beginning to nurse.

Apply ice for a few minutes before feeding to improve nipple erection.

Use electric or hand pump to cause nipple prominence, express a few drops of breast milk, then switch to regular nursing.

Inadequate Letdown

Massage breasts before nursing.

Feed in a quiet, private place, away from distraction.

Take a warm shower before nursing to relax and stimulate letdown.

Apply warm pack for 20 minutes before nursing.

Use relaxation techniques and focus on letdown.

Drink water, juice, or noncaffeinated beverages before and during feeding.

Avoid overfatigue by resting when the baby sleeps, feeding while lying down, and having quiet time alone.

Develop a conditioned response by establishing a routine for starting feedings.

Allow the baby sufficient time (at least 10–15 minutes per side) to trigger the letdown reflex.

Use breast-alternating method (either use different breast for each feeding or switch breasts several times during a single feeding).

If all else fails, obtain a prescription for oxytocin nasal spray from the healthcare provider.

Nipple Soreness

Ensure that infant is correctly positioned at the breast with the infant's ear, shoulder, and hip in straight alignment.

Use finger to break suction before removing infant from the breast.

Hold baby close when feeding to avoid undue pulling on nipple.

Do not allow baby to sleep with nipple in mouth.

Nurse more frequently.

Begin nursing on less-sore breast.

Apply ice to nipples and areola for a few minutes before feeding.

Protect nipples to prevent skin breakdown.

Clean nipple gently with warm water.

Allow nipples to air dry, dry nipples with hair dryer set on low heat, or expose nipples to sunlight initially for 30 seconds, then increase to 3 minutes.

Table 9–2　Self-Care Measures for the Woman with Breast-Feeding Problems (continued)

If clothing rubs nipples, use ventilated shields to keep clothing away from skin.

To promote healing, apply a small amount of breast milk to nipple and areola after nursing and allow to dry.

The routine application of ointment to nipple, areola, or breast (e.g., lanolin, Masse cream, Eucerin cream, or A and D ointment) should be discouraged.

Apply tea bags soaked in warm water.

Change breast pads frequently.

Nurse long enough to empty breasts completely.

Alternate breasts several times during feedings.

Cracked Nipples

Use interventions discussed under Sore Nipples section.

Inspect nipples carefully for cracks or fissures.

Temporarily stop nursing on the affected breast and hand express milk for a day or two until cracks heal.

Maintain healthy diet. Protein and vitamin C are essential for healing.

Use a mild p.o. analgesic such as acetaminophen for discomfort 20–30 minutes before feedings.

Consult healthcare provider if signs of infection develop.

Nipple shield should be tried before nursing on a breast is permanently discontinued, but it should be used only as a last resort. Some women find it contributes to their discomfort. Consult a lactation specialist prior to use.

Breast Engorgement

Nurse frequently (every 1½–3 hours) around the clock.

Wear a well-fitting, supportive bra at all times.

Take a warm shower or apply warm compresses to trigger letdown.

Massage breasts and then hand-express some milk to soften the breast so the infant can "latch on."

Breast-feed long enough to empty breast.

Alternate starting breast.

Take a mild analgesic 20 minutes before feeding if discomfort is pronounced.

Plugged Ducts (Caked Breasts)

Nurse frequently and for long enough to empty the breasts completely.

Rotate feeding position.

Massage breasts before feeding, in a warm shower when possible.

Maintain good nutrition and adequate fluid intake.

- Review signs of illness or problems that need to be referred to the healthcare provider.
- Talk with the parents to determine if they have questions about resuming sexual activity and if they desire information regarding contraceptive measures (see Chapters 7 and 8 for additional information).

BREAST-FEEDING CONCERNS FOLLOWING DISCHARGE

Because of early discharge before breast-feeding is well established, the nurse during the home visit is in a unique position to positively impact the success of breast-feeding (Association of Women's Health, Obstetric and Neonatal Nurses [AWHONN], 2006). Table 9–2 summarizes self-care measures the nurse can suggest to the woman with a breast-feeding problem.

REFERENCES

American Academy of Pediatrics (AAP), Committee on Fetus and Newborn & American College of Obstetricians and Gynecologists (ACOG) Committee on Obstetrics. (2007). *Guidelines for perinatal care* (6th ed.). Evanston, IL: Author.

American Academy of Pediatrics Task Force on Sudden Infant Death Syndrome. (2005). The changing concept of sudden infant death syndrome: diagnostic coding shifts, controversies regarding the sleeping environment, and new variables to consider in reducing risk. *Pediatrics, 116*(5), 1245–1255.

Association of Women's Health, Obstetrical, and Neonatal Nurses (AWHONN). (2006). *The compendium of postpartum care.* Washington, DC: Author.

10 THE AT-RISK POSTPARTAL CLIENT

POSTPARTAL HEMORRHAGE

- Postpartal hemorrhage is caused by uterine atony (relaxation of uterus due to overdistention of uterus, preeclampsia, intra-amniotic infusion, use of magnesium sulfate in labor); retained placental fragments; laceration of genital tract; and vulvar, vaginal, or subperitoneal hematomas and coagulation disorders.
- It is characterized by bright-red vaginal bleeding in the presence of either a soft boggy uterus with clots or a well-contracted uterus without clots.
- Early (primary) hemorrhage commonly occurs within the first 24 hours after giving birth. Late (secondary) hemorrhage occurs after 24 hours to 6 weeks after birth.

Management of Postpartal Hemorrhage

- **Uterine atony.** Oxytocic drugs are administered after separation of the placenta to prevent uterine atony. Methylergonovine maleate (Methergine) intramuscularly (IM) (see Drug Guide: Methylergonovine Maleate, pp. 298–299) or intravenous (IV) oxytocin (see Drug Guide: Oxytocin [Pitocin], pp. 303–307) may be ordered for immediate management of uterine atony. Fundal height and firmness are determined; if the uterus is not firm and well contracted after expulsion of the placenta, fundal massage is initiated. If there is excessive bleeding, the clinician may do bimanual uterine compression or use a balloon tamponade to control bleeding. Hematocrit (Hct) and hemoglobin are monitored. Prostaglandins

10

(IM or directly injected into the uterine cavity) may be used after failed attempts to control bleeding with oxytocic agents.

- **Retained placental fragments.** Inspect the placenta for any signs that a cotyledon or piece of placental membrane is missing. If missing pieces are suspected, the uterine cavity requires uterine exploration and manual removal of tissue. Sonography may be considered to look for retained fragments. Methylergonovine maleate (Methergine) IM or orally (see Drug Guide) is ordered.

- **Lacerations.** Genital tract lacerations should be suspected when vaginal bleeding persists in the presence of a firmly contracted uterus. A visual examination of the cervix is made, and deep cervical lacerations are sutured to stop the bleeding.

- **Hematomas.** Hematomas present as severe pressure or pain anywhere along the genital tract and purple color to the vaginal mucosa or ecchymotic perineum. Small hematomas are managed with ice packs, analgesia, and ongoing observation. They usually reabsorb naturally. Larger hematomas or those increasing in size are incised, and drained to achieve hemostasis. Bleeding vessels are ligated. Vaginal packing may or may not be inserted to achieve hemostasis if needed. Large vaginal packs can make voiding difficult, and an indwelling catheter is often necessary. Because incision and drainage may predispose the woman to infection, broad-spectrum antibiotics are ordered.

Nursing Assessments for Postpartum Hemorrhage

- Assess blood pressure (BP), pulse, and respirations per postpartum agency protocol. If vaginal bleeding is noted, assess BP, pulse, and respirations every 15 minutes.

Be alert for hypotension and tachycardia, which can be signs of hypovolemia, along with tachypnea, decreased BP, pallor, cyanosis, cold and clammy skin, and restlessness. A deceptive feature of postpartal hemorrhage is that maternal vital signs may not change until significant blood loss has occurred because of the increased blood volume associated with pregnancy.

- Assess fundal status for height and firmness (see Procedures: Assessing the Status of the Uterine Fundus after Birth, pp. 318–321). Uterus should be firm and at or below the umbilicus. A well-contracted fundus rules out uterine atony.

- Assess amount of blood loss/vaginal bleeding and any blood clots expressed. **Assessment technique:** Visual assessment; do pad counts within a given time period or weigh the perineal pads (1 mL of blood weighs 1 g).

Be alert for blood loss. To determine the amount of blood loss, assess not only the peripads but also the underpads for pooling of blood. To do so, have the woman turn on her side.

- Examine perineum and buttocks for discoloration, bulging, tender areas. If woman is still recovering from regional anesthesia, frequent visualization of perineum/buttocks is essential. Palpate obvious masses for tenderness and fluctuation.

- Examine vagina or rectum for protruding masses. **Assessment technique:** Position woman on her side, raise her upper buttock, and instruct her to bear down.

Be alert for bulging purplish mass that may become apparent at the introitus, or a soft mass, which may be palpable upon rectal exam.

- Assess women's pain level. After effects of anesthesia have subsided, vaginal and vulvar hematomas are associated with perineal pain or rectal pressure, often intense and out of proportion to what seems apparent in the area.

- Assess for bladder distention (hinders effective uterine contractions and involution process).

- Assess intake and output every 8 hours. *Be alert for* urine output; it needs to stay at greater than 30 mL/hr to perfuse kidneys well.
- Assess laboratory results. *Be alert for* decreasing Hct and notify CNM/ physician if a 10-point decrease in Hct.
- Assess woman's coping responses, level of understanding of her condition, and emotional status.
- Assess woman's ability to take care of her baby because of fatigue related to blood loss. Also assess existing support systems at home.

Sample Nursing Diagnoses
- *Deficient fluid volume* related to blood loss secondary to uterine atony, retained placental fragments, lacerations, or hematoma formation
- *Risk for infection* related to trauma and hemorrhage

Nursing Interventions for Postpartum Hemorrhage
- Gently massage boggy uterus while supporting lower uterine segment (see Figure 10–1) to stimulate contraction and express clots. *Be alert for* level of massage. Forceful

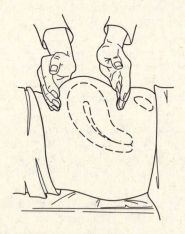

Figure 10–1 ■ Uterine massage.

massage can tire the uterus, resulting in uterine atony, and can cause pain. Be gentle. Do not be misled by the fact that a woman has a firm uterus. Significant bleeding can occur from causes other than uterine atony.

- Monitor type and amount of bleeding and associated consistency of the uterus. *Be alert for* dark-red blood and relaxed uterus, which indicate uterine atony or retained placental fragments. Bright-red vaginal bleeding and contracted uterus indicate laceration hemorrhage.

- Apply ice pack during first hour after birth for women at risk for vaginal hematoma. If hematoma forms, use sitz bath after 12 hours.

- Maintain IV for fluid maintenance, especially if frequent fundal massage has been necessary. Start second IV with an 18-gauge needle to administer blood products if necessary. Send blood for type and cross match if not already done in the birthing area. Assess consistency of fundus and the presence of normal versus excessive lochia before discontinuing the IV.

- Administer oxytocics per order. Carefully note uterine tone and BP response to medication.

- Monitor intake and output hourly. Initially insert Foley catheter to ensure accurate output determination.

- Administer pain medications for discomfort as ordered.

- Provide stool or chair for use during shower in case of dizziness or weakness to facilitate self-care and progressive ambulation.

- Review the following critical aspects of the care you have provided:

  1. Have I effectively monitored her fundal and lochia status? Did I quickly identify and intervene when there was continued relaxation of the uterus and expression of clots? Did I carry out the uterine massage as gently as possible?

  2. Are the woman's vital signs stable? Is the woman showing any signs of hypovolemia?

  3. Is the woman complaining of discomfort anywhere along the genital tract? Have I provided adequate

comfort measures for her, such as cold or warm packs, perineal care, sitz baths, or pain medication?

4. Have I assisted in decreasing the anxiety of the woman and her family by keeping them informed about her status?

5. Have I provided the mother with home care information on the following: iron supplementation, expected changes in fundus and lochia, how to massage the fundus as indicated by tone, signs of abnormal bleeding, and when to call a healthcare provider?

Evaluation

- Signs of postpartal hemorrhage are detected quickly and managed effectively.
- Hematoma formation is detected quickly and managed successfully.
- The woman's discomfort is relieved effectively.
- The woman is able to identify abnormal changes that might occur following discharge and understands the importance of notifying her caregiver if they develop.
- Maternal-infant attachment is maintained successfully.

SUBINVOLUTION (LATE [SECONDARY] POSTPARTAL HEMORRHAGE)

- Subinvolution is defined as failure of the uterus to follow the normal pattern of involution.
- Signs and symptoms of subinvolution are not usually apparent until about 4–6 weeks postpartum. The fundus remains higher in the abdomen/pelvis than expected. Lochia often fails to progress from rubra to serosa to alba. The lochia may remain rubra or return to rubra several days postpartum. Lochia rubra that persists longer than 2 weeks postpartum is highly suggestive of subinvolution. The amount of lochia may be more profuse than expected. Leukorrhea, backache, and foul lochia may occur if infection is present. The woman may also relate a history of irregular or excessive bleeding after the birth.

- Late postpartal hemorrhage is less common but can be extremely stressful for the woman and her family, who are at home by this time.

Management of Subinvolution

- **Uterine examination.** Bimanual uterine exam shows an enlarged, softer-than-normal uterus.
- **Drug therapy.** Oral methylergonovine 0.2 mg or ergonovine 0.2 mg q3–4h for 24–48 hours is given to stimulate uterine contractility (see Drug Guide: Methylergonovine Maleate [Methergine], pp. 298–299). Oral antibiotics are ordered if metritis (infection) is present or invasive procedures are done.
- **Uterine curettage.** If treatment is not effective or if retained placental fragments and polyps are the cause, curettage may be done.

Nursing Assessments for Subinvolution

- Assess characteristics of lochial pattern since birth. *Be alert for* lochia pattern: lochia that does not progress from rubra to serosa or returns to rubra days after the birth.
- Assess whether mother has felt feverish or has had a temperature. *Be alert for* elevation in temperature, which can occur if infection is the cause of subinvolution.
- Assess woman's level of understanding regarding her condition, the signs of subinvolution, and when she should call her healthcare provider.

Sample Nursing Diagnoses

- *Acute pain* related to stimulation of uterine contraction secondary to administration of oxytocic medications
- *Risk for infection* related to bacterial invasion of uterus secondary to dilatation and curettage
- *Health-seeking behaviors* related to lack of information about delayed postpartum hemorrhage

Nursing Interventions for Subinvolution

- During discharge teaching, review normal involution process and progression of lochia from rubra to serosa to alba. Stress that the woman should report any continued bleeding that does not go away with rest and medication and that covers the surface of one perineal pad 2–6 weeks after birth. Any adverse effects from the medications should be reported to the healthcare provider.

- Discuss the importance of increasing the length and number of rest periods; see if she can have a support person with her during the 24-hour oxytocic medication period. Refer to home care.
- Inform the lactating woman that she can continue to breast-feed. Low-dose methylergonovine poses no threat to the baby, and breast-feeding can assist in involution.
- If woman has history of elevated BP, teach her the early signs of adverse effects of oxytocic medication on her BP. These signs include nausea, vomiting, headache, and complaints of abdominal cramping or signs of circulatory stasis, including itching, tingling, numbness, and cold fingers and toes.

Sample Nurse's Charting

1930: T 99.2°F, P 92, R 16, BP 124/76. Fundus soft, 1 FB above symphysis pubis and midline. Tender to palpation. Lochia rubra with small clots. Complains of fatigue, lochia flow return to rubra, and soaking surface of one peripad/day 15 days after birth. Is breast-feeding and expresses concern over continued rubra lochia and progressive fatigue. S. Paulski, RNC

Evaluation

- Woman knows the signs of delayed uterine involution and when to report them to her healthcare provider.
- Woman understands the treatment regimen and takes her medications as ordered.
- Woman has support to help her deal with increased fatigue and anxiety related to the failure of uterus to return to normal.

TYPES OF REPRODUCTIVE TRACT INFECTIONS

Type/Cause	Signs/Symptoms	Treatment
Localized Infection of External Genitals Episiotomy or sutured laceration; infected traumatized perineum, vulva, vagina, or abdominal incision	Low-grade fever (38.3°C [101°F]), localized pain, edema, warmth, redness, seropurulent discharge. Late: gaping of previously approximated wound, high temperature.	Oral broad-spectrum antibiotics, sitz bath and surgigator, analgesics, removal of stitches to promote drainage; if abscess forms, use of saline gauze 2–3 times a day to keep lesion open and remove necrotic tissue.
Endometritis (Metritis) Infection of total endometrium or placental site	In severe endometritis cases: Sawtooth fever pattern with fever spikes (101°F [38.3°C] to 103°F [39.4°C]); chills, tachycardia. Tender uterus. Scant to profuse dark-brown, foul-smelling discharge. In β-hemolytic *Streptococcus* infection, scant, serosanguineous, and odorless lochia.	Antibiotics until woman is afebrile for 24–48 hours, oxytocics to stimulate contraction and lochial drainage, semi-Fowler's position and/or ambulation to promote drainage. Aerobic and anaerobic blood, and lochial culture, hydration.

Type/Cause	Signs/Symptoms	Treatment
Parametritis (Pelvic Cellulitis) Infection of tissues around uterus via the lymphatics (often following endometritis)	Marked high fever (102–104°F, [38.9–40°C]), chills, malaise, lethargy, tachycardia, abdominal pain. Local and rebound pain during pelvic exam. Increase incidence of abscesses.	Broad-spectrum antibiotics (intravenous) until the results of culture and sensitivity reports are available. IV antibiotics until woman is afebrile for 48 hrs. Abcesses are seen as palpable mass, confirmed by US. Require I & D to avoid rupture and peritonitis. After drainage, abscess cavity may be packed with iodoform gauze to promote drainage and facilitate healing.

IV, intravenous.

Nursing Assessments for Reproductive Tract Infections

- Assess BP, pulse, and respirations every 2–4 hours. Tachycardia is associated with endometritis and pelvic cellulitis.
- Assess temperature every 4 hours unless elevated, then every 2 hours.

  Tip: Remember that a low-grade fever is common during the first 24 hours after birth. Be alert for elevated temperature (greater than 100.4°F [38°C]) patterns.

- Assess fundal height, tone, and sensation (see Procedures: Assessing the Status of the Uterine Fundus

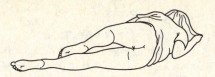

Figure 10–2 Episiotomy is inspected. Woman is on her side, and her upper leg is forward.

after Birth pp. 318–321). Note any discomfort or pain that is greater than anticipated and note protracted afterpains.

- Assess perineum every 8 hours. Inspect perineum using good light source. **Assessment technique:** Have woman lie on her side with her top leg slightly forward and ahead of the bottom leg (see Figure 10–2). After donning disposable gloves, lift the buttock to expose the perineum and the anus. If no episiotomy is present, the perineum is described as intact. Assess episiotomy or sutured laceration for redness, edema, ecchymosis, discharge, approximation of edges (skin edges together) [REEDA scale], and tenderness.

- Assess lochia for type, amount, and odor (see Procedures: Evaluating Lochia, pp. 327–330).

- Assess laboratory results for above normal postpartum levels, especially the white blood cell count.

   Tip: Normal postpartum leukocyte levels are already increased (15,000–30,000/mm^3), so be alert for greater than 30,000/mm^3.

- Assess hydration status.

- Assess for abscess formation (often a palpable mass and fever).

Sample Nursing Diagnoses

- *Risk for infection* related to broken skin or traumatized tissues
- *Acute pain* related to the presence of infection
- *Altered parenting* related to mother's malaise and other symptoms of infection

Nursing Interventions for Reproductive Tract Infections

- Monitor temperature every 4 hours and identify trends. *Be alert for* low-grade fever (101°F [38.3°C]) with rapid onset, which indicates localized infection. Irregular fever (sawtooth pattern), varying from 101–103°F (38.3–39.4°C) indicates endometritis. Persistent high fever (102–104°F [38.9–40°C]) and chills indicate parametritis.

- Monitor lochial changes for signs of failure of normal involution.

- Teach woman about, and perform, proper perineal and hygienic measures to promote healing and prevent contamination of the perineum, such as washing hands frequently and after each peripad change, perineal care (see Chapter 7), and use of sitz bath or surgigator. Encourage a diet high in protein and vitamin C.

- Teach woman with draining wound or purulent lochia about wound care and proper management of soiled dressings and linen.

- Obtain cultures of lochia, wound, and urine (to rule out asymptomatic urinary tract infection [UTI]).

  Tip: With episiotomy infections, lochia may have a foul odor and appear yellow.

- Administer antibiotics, oxytocics (see Drug Guide: Oxytocin [Pitocin], pp. 303–307, and Drug Guide: Methylergonovine Maleate [Methergine], pp. 298–299) and analgesic spray as prescribed. Instruct on need to take entire course of prescribed medications at home.

- Assist mothers with endometritis to ambulate and lie in semi-Fowler's position to facilitate lochial drainage.

- If parametritis occurs, provide bed rest and maintain IV fluids. Monitor intake and output and urine specific gravity.

- Institute home care referral as needed.

- Maintain mother–infant interaction. Assist mother to balance her need for rest and her need for time with her baby.

Evaluation

- The infection is quickly identified and treated successfully without further complications.
- The woman understands the infection and the purpose of therapy; she carries out any ongoing antibiotic therapy if indicated following discharge.
- Maternal–infant attachment is maintained.

POSTPARTAL THROMBOEMBOLIC DISEASE

- Thromboembolic disease refers primarily to superficial thrombophlebitis (thrombus due to inflammation), which primarily forms in saphenous veins, appears on the 3rd or 4th postpartal day, and shows clinical improvement within 48 hours of therapy.
- Superficial thrombophlebitis often presents as some local heat and redness, mild calf pain, visible and palpable veins, and normal temperature or low-grade fever.
- Deep vein thrombosis (DVT) is seen in women with a history of thrombosis and increases the likelihood of pulmonary emboli development. DVT may present with severe leg pain of sudden onset (pain may worsen if leg is in a dependent position and if pressure is applied to calf area), edema and paleness of affected leg, systemic signs of elevated temperature, pulse and chills, and possible positive Homans' sign. It may take up to 4–6 weeks to resolve after the acute symptoms stop.

Management of Thromboembolic Disease

- **Superficial thrombophlebitis.** Bed rest with leg elevation is ordered. Mist heat therapy is applied to facilitate drainage and decrease venous stasis. Elastic support hose are to be worn after acute inflammation subsides.
- **Deep vein thrombosis.** In addition to treatment for superficial thrombophlebitis, anticoagulant therapy is ordered. Administer heparin using an infusion pump. The desired prothrombin time lab value reaches 1.5–2.0, then sodium warfarin (Coumadin) is begun.

No aspirin or ibuprofen should be taken by women on anticoagulant therapy. The woman may be placed on antibiotic therapy.

Nursing Assessments for Thromboembolic Disease

- Assess vital signs, especially oral temperature, every 4 hours. Be alert for and report temperature greater than 100.4°F.
- Assess calves, thighs, and groin area (especially left side) bilaterally for increase in size, color, warmth, peripheral pulses, and positive Homans' sign. **Assessment technique for Homans' sign:** Dorsiflex foot with knee in extended position (see Figure 10–3). If pain occurs in foot or leg with foot dorsiflexion, Homans' sign is positive.
- Assess complete blood cell count, platelet count, and prothrombin time.
- Assess for evidence of bleeding related to heparin therapy.

Sample Nursing Diagnoses

- *Ineffective tissue perfusion in periphery* related to obstructed venous stasis
- *Altered tissue perfusion* related to pulmonary embolism secondary to dislodgement of deep vein thrombus

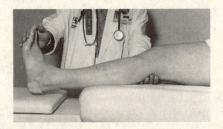

Figure 10–3 ■ Homans' sign: With the woman's knee flexed to decrease the risk of embolization, the nurse dorsiflexes the foot. Pain in the foot or leg is a positive Homans' sign.

Nursing Interventions
for Thromboembolic Disease

- Monitor vital signs. *Be alert for* elevated temperature, which may be associated with inflammation.
- Inspect and palpate calf, thigh, and groin area daily for heat, color, tenderness, and peripheral pulses. *Be alert for* increasing redness, swelling, or pain.
- Monitor any signs of DVT. *Be alert for* sudden onset of severe leg or thigh pain, elevated temperature, or chills. Report these signs to physician immediately.
- Measure affected portion of leg with nonstretch tape to assess degree of edema.
- Assist mother to stay on bed rest with her leg fully elevated on pillows. Do not use knee gatch on bed and avoid any pressure on popliteal space (to prevent pelvic pooling and impedance of blood flow). While mother is on bed rest, have her use footboard, do passive exercises, and change position frequently.
- Apply warm, moist packs to affected leg (vasodilatation facilitates blood flow and decreases pain). Be sure to wrap packs to prevent burns and remove for 10 minutes each hour.
- Administer antibiotics per order.
- Administer heparin as ordered after obtaining prothrombin results. Monitor prothrombin and Hct to evaluate bleeding and adequacy of heparinization.

  Special alert: One percent protamine sulfate is used as the antidote for heparin overdose.
- Initiate progressive ambulation after acute inflammation subsides.
- Apply support hose (compresses superficial veins and increases deep venous flow).
- Monitor and report signs of pulmonary emboli. *Be alert for* signs such as vague chest pain, anxiety, respiratory rate greater than 16 breaths per minute, pallor, tachypnea, and possible changes in lung sounds (rales and friction rub).

- Instruct mother on measures to prevent venous stasis:
  1. Avoid crossing legs at the knee while sitting and elevate the feet while sitting when possible.
  2. Avoid prolonged standing or sitting.
  3. Ambulate periodically throughout the day.
  4. Drink at least six 8-oz glasses of water per day.
- Instruct mother regarding anticoagulant therapy:
  1. Take medication at the same time each day.
  2. Keep appointments so that clotting times can be monitored and medication can be adjusted.
  3. Be aware of signs of heparin overdose such as bleeding gums, ecchymosis, nosebleed, hematuria, and melena.
  4. Note any blood in the stools; it should be reported to the physician.
  5. Maintain current eating habits (include green vegetables) and lifestyle.
  6. Wear a MedicAlert bracelet indicating use of anti-coagulants.
  7. Avoid any activities that may cause bleeding, such as playing contact sports, using stiff toothbrushes, or shaving legs with a straight razor.
  8. Avoid medications such as aspirin and nonsteroidal antiinflammatory drugs that increase anticoagulant activity.
  9. Avoid herbals such as garlic, ginger, and ginkgo, which prolong prothrombin time, and excessive amounts of vitamins K, C, and E that affect coagulation.
  10. Report results of home testing for thromboplastin-mediated clotting factors.
- If woman wishes to continue breast-feeding, have her discuss use of low-dose subcutaneous heparin at home or warfarin.
- Review the following critical aspects of the care you have provided:

1. Have I administered the correct dose of heparin at the designated times after first reviewing the results of the clotting studies?
2. Have I been alert for any signs of heparin overdose?
3. What can I do to assist the woman to maintain bed rest?
4. Is the mother able to eat a diet that assists her coagulation status?
5. Have I assessed the woman's understanding of her thrombolic status and answered her questions? Have I given her opportunities to practice preventive measures?

- Review with the couple the signs and symptoms of thrombophlebitis and the need to report them since the condition may not occur until after discharge. *Tip:* Do not massage affected leg.

Evaluation

- If thrombosis or thrombophlebitis develops, it is detected quickly and managed without further complications.
- At discharge, the woman is able to explain the purpose, dosage regimen, and necessary precautions associated with any prescribed medications such as anticoagulants.
- The woman can discuss self-care measures and ongoing therapies (such as the use of elastic stockings) that are indicated.
- The woman has bonded successfully with her newborn and is able to care for the baby effectively.

POSTPARTUM URINARY TRACT INFECTION (UTI)

- Typically, this infection is caused by gram-negative organisms such as *Escherichia coli*, which invade the urethra and bladder and cause cystitis. Bladder bacteria then may ascend to the kidney as a result of vesicoureteral reflux during voiding, causing pyelonephritis after several days.

- Postpartal women are at increased risk because of decreased bladder sensitivity due to stretching, trauma, and retention of residual urine; bacteria introduced during catheterization; and bladder trauma during childbirth.
- Women may present with dysuria, urinary urgency and frequency, suprapubic or lower abdominal pain, lower back discomfort, and possibly hematuria.
- In addition to the signs and symptoms of cystitis, pyelonephritis presents as cloudy urine and systemic signs of high fever, chills, nausea and vomiting (N&V), malaise, fatigue, severe flank pain, and costovertebral angle tenderness (CVAT). Cystitis management must continue after symptoms disappear, because this infection tends to recur.

Management of Postpartal Urinary Tract Infection

- **Urinalysis.** Urinalysis is obtained and analyzed for protein, blood, and organisms. Urine that contains an increase in white blood cells (WBCs) (greater than 100,000/mL organisms) and protein and/or blood indicates UTI. Urine culture and sensitivities are obtained so organism-specific antibiotics can be identified.
- **Fluid and drug management.** Fluid intake is increased to 3–4 L/day to dilute the urine and initiate flushing out of the infected urine. Therapeutic doses of vitamin C or cranberry juice are used to acidify the urine. Urine acidification decreases bacterial growth and increases the action of urinary tract antiseptics. Short-acting sulfonamides such as nitrofurantoin (Macrobid) are ordered except in term pregnancy, when sulfamethoxazole-trimethoprim (Septra-DS, Bactrim-DS) may be given. In case of sulfa allergy, ampicillin or amoxicillin-clavulanic acid (Augmentin) can be used for 7–10 days. Antispasmodics or urinary analgesics, such as phenazopyridine hydrochloride (Pyridium), may be given to relieve discomfort.

- **Pyelonephritis management.** If woman develops pyelonephritis, she may be hospitalized for aggressive treatment and monitoring to prevent permanent kidney damage. IV medications are given, and an indwelling bladder catheter may be put in place. Relief of symptoms is usually obtained in 24–48 hours.

Nursing Assessments for Postpartal Urinary Tract Infections

- Assess bladder function for frequency, urgency, and amount of urine output. Inspect urine for color (hematuria), odor, and appearance (concentrated or dilute).
- Assess for painful or burning urination.
- Assess for increased vaginal bleeding, boggy uterus, and uterine cramping.
- Palpate for large mass, at or near umbilicus, which displaces uterine fundus upward, denoting an overdistended bladder.
- Assess for complaints of suprapubic or lower abdominal discomfort, lower back pain, or severe flank pain.
- Palpate for costovertebral tenderness.
- Assess vital signs q4h and observe for signs of systemic involvement.
- Assess intake and output q8h.

Sample Nursing Diagnoses

- *Urinary retention* related to decreased bladder sensitivity and normal postpartal diuresis
- *Risk for infection* related to urinary stasis secondary to overdistention
- *Health-seeking behaviors* related to lack of information about UTI, its treatment, and its possible sequelae

Nursing Interventions for Postpartal Urinary Tract Infections

- Assist woman to obtain clean-catch, midstream sample for urinalysis to prevent contamination with lochia.

- Encourage woman to void q2–4h and empty bladder completely. Pouring warm water over the perineum or having the woman void in a sitz bath may be effective. Provide ice pack for perineum within 1 hour after birth to decrease edema formation and facilitate voiding.
- Woman should drink at least eight to ten 8-oz glasses of liquids, especially water, each day. Also encourage woman to drink unsweetened cranberry, plum, apricot, or prune juices, which increase acidity of urine. Avoid carbonated beverages.
- Provide comfort measures, such as back massage, and analgesics for back and flank pain, antispasmodics for dysuria and cramping, antiemetics for N&V, and oral hygiene to promote comfort. If woman has a fever, provide tepid baths and antipyretics.
- If woman is taking sulfonamide drugs, instruct her that breast-feeding may be discontinued and teach her how to pump her breasts.

Be alert for use of sulfonamides. These medications are secreted in breast milk and combine with proteins to create neonatal jaundice; therefore, pumped milk should be discarded while mother is taking these medications.

- Monitor baby for diarrhea and yeast infections (candidiasis) while mother is taking ampicillin.
- Instruct mother that her urine may change color with prescribed medication.

Be alert for the following: Azo Gantrisin can turn urine red or red orange; nitrofurantoin creates brown urine, may cause N&V and diarrhea, and should be taken with food or milk to decrease gastric irritation.

- Reinforce instruction on prophylactic hygienic practice (e.g., wiping from front to back, voiding when she feels the urge to void, wearing cotton underclothing, and voiding after intercourse). Encourage woman to drink two glasses of water immediately after intercourse to increase urine output and flush out contaminants that may have entered the urethra.

Evaluation

- Woman understands any special instructions for taking medications and need for follow-up urine culture.
- Woman knows hygienic, nutritional, and fluid requirements to avoid UTIs and any symptoms to report to healthcare provider.

MASTITIS

Inflammation of the breast commonly is caused by *Staphylococcus aureus*, *Haemophilus parainfluenzae*, or *H. influenzae* from the infant's nose and throat, hands of the mother, or birthing unit personnel. Contributing factors include clogged milk ducts, lowered maternal defenses due to fatigue or stress, unclean hands, and cracked or fissured nipples. *Candida albicans* is another cause. This usually occurs in the 2nd or 4th week postpartum. A breast abscess may be a complication.

Management of Mastitis

- **Drug therapy.** Antibiotics are ordered for a full 10-day course, even if symptoms subside within a few days. For *Candida* infections, use of topical antifungals is indicated. Antipyretics, such as acetaminophen and nonsteroidal antiinflammatory agents, are used to treat fever and inflammation.
- **Breast-feeding.** Continued breast-feeding is recommended. In the presence of a yeast infection, the mother and baby are both treated with antifungals.
- **Laboratory tests.** Culture the breast milk and look for elevated leukocyte and bacterial counts.
- **Breast abscess management.** If a breast abscess forms, the breast milk and any drainage are cultured. The abscessed area may be aspirated or incised and drained.

Nursing Assessments for Mastitis

- Examine breast for localized redness, tenderness, and swelling. On palpation, it may be very hard and hot, and the lump may feel like a hard mothball.

- Inspect nipple for fissures or cracks (entry points for infection). *Be alert for* inflamed and painful nipples, which may indicate a yeast or fungus infection. Breast abscesses appear as hardened, painful local areas of inflammation below the skin surface.
- Assess mother's general physical status. Systemic symptoms include flulike symptoms: headache, malaise, muscle ache, rapid pulse, and temperature of about 38.5°C (101.3°F).
- Assess mother's dietary and sleep patterns and level of stress. Decreases in dietary intake and sleep and/or excessive stress and activity can decrease mother's resistance to infection.
- Assess feeding history for precipitating factors such as ineffective emptying of breasts, engorgement, breast compression from tight clothing or bra, or sudden change in feeding pattern, such as baby sleeping through the night or use of supplemental feedings.
- Inspect baby's mouth for white patches surrounded by redness on the buccal membrane, which indicate presence of *Candida albicans*, or thrush.

Sample Nursing Diagnoses
- *Health-seeking behaviors* related to lack of information about appropriate breast-feeding practices
- *Risk for infection* related to cracked and traumatized breast tissue or nipples
- *Ineffective breast-feeding* related to pain secondary to development of mastitis

Nursing Interventions for Mastitis
Preventive Measures
- Discuss predisposing factors.
- Use good hand-washing technique.
- Instruct mother about breast care: hand-washing before handling breasts or nipples, cleansing of breast with water only (to maintain protective oils), wearing

supportive bra at all times (to avoid milk stasis in lower lobes), and changing bra and breast pads frequently.
- Reinforce mother's knowledge about breast-feeding techniques, such as position, frequency, and removal of baby from breast.
- Provide special attention to mothers who have blocked milk ducts, which increase the risk for mastitis.

If the Woman Has Mastitis

- Administer antifungals as ordered and pain medications usually before feeding to ease discomfort.
- Teach mother to increase feeding frequency, increase fluid intake (six to eight 8-oz glasses a day), be on bed rest for first 24 hours, have friends or relatives assist with care in order to increase rest periods, breast-feed first on unaffected breast until letdown occurs (promotes complete emptying of both breasts), express milk at least every 3 hours, and massage caked areas toward nipple during feeding (see Figure 10–4).
- Mother's temperature should be monitored every 4 hours until infection resolves.
- Instruct mother that if there is no improvement within 12–14 hours or if fever persists, she should notify her healthcare provider. If mother is on antibiotics and the baby develops diarrhea, she should let her physician know.
- Provide support if mother needs to discontinue breast-feeding temporarily and instruct her on expression of milk.

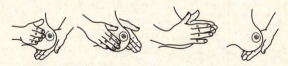

Figure 10–4 ■ Breast massage. Caked areas of breast are massaged toward the nipple.

Evaluation

- The mother is able to identify predisposing factors, signs and symptoms of impending mastitis, and preventive measures.
- Mother knows proper management if mastitis occurs. Mother is supported in her decision to breast-feed and knows how to resume if it is necessary to stop.

ONGOING MANAGEMENT OF SELECTED PERINATAL COMPLICATIONS

Preeclampsia

The postpartum goal is to prevent eclamptic seizures and neurologic sequelae.

Effect of Postpartum on Preeclampsia	Critical Nursing Interventions
Postpartum diuresis decreases serum magnesium sulfate levels, thereby increasing the possibility of seizures.	Monitor vital signs (VS) closely for 48 hours after birth (vital signs should remain stable then begin to slowly decrease). Monitor urine output (less than 30 mL/hr) and deep tendon reflexes (DTRs). Administer intravenous magnesium sulfate for 24 hours after birth. Check urine for protein and specific gravity qhr. Administer diuretic as ordered. Do not give oxytocics because of their hypertensive properties. Minimize environmental stimuli until status improves. Have seizure precautions in place.

Effect of Postpartum on Preeclampsia	**Critical Nursing Interventions**
Magnesium sulfate causes uterine relaxation, which increases the possibility of uterine atony; preeclampsia decreases blood volume and lowers platelet counts, which can lead to postpartum hemorrhage.	Monitor for signs of postpartum hemorrhage. Carefully massaging the uterus is important. Encourage frequent voiding to keep bladder empty and avoid uterine atony. Emotional support is essential during critical illnesses.

Diabetes

The goal is to maintain normal blood glucose levels, prevent postpartum complications (preeclampsia, hemorrhage, infection), and enhance parent–infant interaction.

Effect of Postpartum on Diabetes	**Critical Nursing Interventions**
Loss of placental insulin inhibitory hormone (human chorionic somatomammotropin [hCS], progesterone) drops insulin requirement sharply. Some women do not require insulin for the first day or so. Increased use of glucose during postpartum.	Draw blood glucose sample immediately after birth. Monitor urine for glucose and ketone q2h × 24 hours. Administer insulin on sliding scale based on blood or urine glucose test per physician order. Monitor for hypoglycemia (see Chapter 2). Maintain intravenous (IV) glucose for 24 hours after birth then restart diabetic diet.
Increased postpartum complications, such as preeclampsia.	Monitor vital signs for at least 48 hours. Be alert for preeclampsia symptoms (see Chapter 2).

Effect of Postpartum on Diabetes	Critical Nursing Interventions
Hemorrhage due to uterine atony and increased amniotic fluid.	Monitor uterine involution.
Any infection complicates diabetic regulation and increases risk of acidosis.	Maintain excellent hand-washing for self. Stress personal hygiene to avoid infections.
Altered parent–infant interaction because baby requires special observation.	Promote flexible visiting policy. Keep parents informed of baby's progress and status. If mother is breast-feeding, have her increase her caloric intake by 400–500 kcal/day (20% protein); adjust insulin dosage as needed per physician order. Provide for pumping or breast-feeding opportunities q2–4h around the clock.

Drug Guide

Betamethasone (Celestone Soluspan)

Overview of Maternal-Fetal Action

Studies have provided ample evidence that glucocorticoids such as betamethasone are capable of inducing pulmonary maturation and decreasing the incidence of respiratory distress syndrome in preterm infants. The mechanism by which corticosteroids accelerate fetal lung maturity is unclear, but it is related to the stimulation of enzyme activity by the drug. The enzyme is required for biosynthesis of surfactant by the type II pneumocytes. Surfactant is of major importance to the proper functioning of the lung in that it decreases the surface tension of the alveoli. Glucocorticoids also increase the rate of glycogen depletion, which leads to thinning of the interalveolar septa and increases the size of the alveoli. The thinning of the epithelium brings the capillaries into closer proximity with the air spaces and improves oxygen exchange.

Route, Dosage, Frequency

Prenatal maternal intramuscular injections of 12 mg of betamethasone are given once a day for 2 days. Dexamethasone has also been given in doses of 6 mg every 12 hours for four doses (Iams & Romero, 2007). To obtain maximum results, birth should be delayed for at least 24 hours after completing the first round of treatment. The effect of corticosteroids may be transient. Repeat courses of corticosteroids should not be used routinely (Gibbs, 2008).

Contraindications

Inability to delay birth

Adequate L/S ratio

Presence of a condition that necessitates immediate birth (e.g., maternal bleeding)

Presence of maternal infection, diabetes mellitus (relative contraindication)

Gestational age greater than 34 completed weeks

Maternal Side Effects

Increased risk for infection has not been supported in large studies. There may, however, be some increase in the incidence of infection in women with premature rupture of the membranes. Maternal hyperglycemia may occur during corticosteroid administration. Insulin-dependent diabetics may require insulin infusions for several days to prevent ketoacidosis. Corticosteroids may possibly increase the risk of pulmonary edema, especially when used concurrently with tocolytics (Briggs, Freeman, & Yaffee, 2005).

Effects on Fetus/Newborn

Lowered cortisol levels at birth, but rebound occurs by 2 hours of age

Hypoglycemia

Increased risk of neonatal sepsis

Animal studies have shown serious fetal side effects, such as reduced head circumference and decreased placental weight. Human studies have not shown these effects, however (Briggs et al., 2005).

Nursing Considerations

- Assess for presence of contraindications.
- Provide education regarding possible side effects.
- Administer betamethasone deep into gluteal muscle, avoiding injection into deltoid (high incidence of local atrophy). (Dexamethasone may be administered IM or IV.)
- Periodically evaluate BP, pulse, weight, and edema.

- Assess lab data for electrolytes and blood glucose.
- Although concomitant use of betamethasone and to-colytic agents has been implicated in increased risk of pulmonary edema, the betamethasone has little mineral corticoid activity; therefore, it probably doesn't add significantly to the salt and water retention effects of betaadrenergic agonists. Other causes of noncardiogenic pulmonary edema should also be investigated if pulmonary edema develops during administration of betamethasone to a woman in preterm labor.

CARBOPROST TROMETHAMINE (HEMABATE)

Overview of Action

Carboprost tromethamine (Hemabate) is used to reduce blood loss secondary to uterine atony. It stimulates myometrial contractions to control postpartum hemorrhaging that is unresponsive to usual techniques. Carboprost tromethamine can also be used to induce labor in women desiring an elective termination of a pregnancy. The drug is also used to induce labor in cases of intrauterine fetal death and hydatidiform mole (Wilson, Shannon, & Shields, 2009).

Pregnancy Risk Category: D

Route, Dosage, Frequency

In cases of immediate postpartum hemorrhage the usual intramuscular dose is 250 mcg (1mL) which can be repeated every 1½ to 3½ hours if uterine atony persists. The dosage can be increased to 500 mcg (2 mL) if uterine contractility is inadequate after several doses of 250 mcg. The total dosage should not exceed 12 mg. The maximum duration of use is 48 hours (Wilson et al., 2009).

Contraindications

The drug is contraindicated in women with active cardiac, pulmonary, or renal disease. It should not be administered during pregnancy or in women with acute pelvic inflammatory disease. It should be used with caution in women with asthma, adrenal disease, hypotension, hypertension, diabetes mellitus, epilepsy, fibroids, cervical stenosis, or previous uterine surgery (Wilson et al., 2009).

Side Effects

The most common side effects are nausea and diarrhea. Fever, chills, and flushing can occur. Headache, muscle, joint, abdominal, or eye pain can also occur (Wilson et al., 2009).

Nursing Considerations

- The injection should be given in a large muscle. Aspiration should be performed to avoid injection into a blood vessel, which can result in bronchospasm, tetanic contractions, and shock.
- After administration, monitor uterine status and bleeding carefully.
- Report excess bleeding to the physician/CNM.
- Check vital signs routinely, observing for an increase in temperature, elevated pulse, and decreased blood pressure.
- Breast-feeding should be delayed for 24 hours after administration (Wilson et al., 2009).

DINOPROSTONE (PREPIDIL) VAGINAL GEL

Overview of Maternal-Fetal Action

Pregnancy Risk Category: C

Dinoprostone is a naturally occurring form of prostaglandin E_2. Dinoprostone can be used at term to ripen the cervix and can stimulate the smooth muscle of the uterus to enhance uterine contractions. Prepidil can be administered endocervically (Pfizer Pharmaceuticals, Inc., 2008).

Route, Dosage, Frequency

The gel contains 0.5 mg of dinoprostone. The gel is placed in the posterior fornix of the vagina, and the client is kept supine for 2 hours, after which time she may ambulate. Continuous electronic monitoring is typically used for 2 hours after administration. Women who show no signs of labor and have a reassuring fetal monitoring strip may be discharged after 2 hours of administration.

Contraindications

- Client with known sensitivity to prostaglandins
- Presence of nonreassuring fetal status
- Unexplained bleeding during pregnancy
- Strong suspicion of cephalopelvic disproportion
- Client already receiving Pitocin
- Client who is not anticipated to be able to give birth vaginally
- Previous cesarean birth, uterine scar, or uterine rupture (Battista & Wing, 2007).

Dinoprostone vaginal gel should be used with **caution** in clients with ruptured membranes, a fetus in breech presentation, presence of glaucoma, or history of asthma (Pfizer Pharmaceuticals, Inc., 2008).

Maternal Side Effects

Uterine hyperstimulation with or without nonreassuring fetal status has occurred in a very small number (6.6%) of clients. Other reported maternal side effects include gastrointestinal disturbance (fewer than 1% of clients have experienced fever, nausea, vomiting, diarrhea, or abdominal pain) (Wilson, Shannon, & Shields, 2009).

Effects on Fetus/Newborn

Nonreassuring fetal heart rate patterns.

Nursing Considerations

- Assess for presence of contraindications.
- Monitor maternal vital signs, cervical dilatation, and effacement carefully.
- Monitor fetal status for presence of reassuring fetal heart rate pattern (baseline 110 to 160 bpm, presence

of variability, presence of accelerations with fetal movement, absence of late or variable decelerations).

- Prepare to administer terbutaline if uterine hyperstimulation, sustained uterine contractions, nonreassuring fetal status, or any other adverse reactions occur.

ERYTHROMYCIN OPHTHALMIC OINTMENT (ILOTYCIN OPHTHALMIC)

Overview of Neonatal Action

Erythromycin (Ilotycin Ophthalmic) is used as prophylactic treatment of ophthalmia neonatorum, which is caused by the bacteria *Neisseria gonorrhoeae*. Preventive treatment of gonorrhea in the newborn is required by law. Erythromycin is also effective against ophthalmic chlamydial infections. It is either bacteriostatic or bactericidal, depending on the organisms involved and the concentration of drug.

Pregnancy Risk Category: B

Route, Dosage, Frequency

Ophthalmic ointment (0.5%) is instilled as a narrow ribbon or strand, 1 cm long, along the lower conjunctival surface of each eye, starting at the inner canthus. It is instilled only once in each eye (AAP & ACOG, 2007). The ointment may be administered in the birthing area or, alternatively, later in the nursery so that eye contact between infant and parent is facilitated and the bonding process immediately after birth is not interrupted. After administration, gently close the eye and manipulate to ensure the spread of ointment (Wilson, Shannon, & Shields, 2009).

Neonatal Side Effects

Sensitivity reaction; may interfere with ability to focus and may cause edema and inflammation. Side effects usually disappear in 24 to 48 hours.

Nursing Considerations

- Wash hands immediately before instillation to prevent introduction of bacteria.
- Do not irrigate the eyes after instillation. Use new tube or single-use container for ophthalmic ointment administration shortly after birth. May wipe away excess after 1 minute with sterile cotton (AAP & ACOG, 2007).
- Observe for hypersensitivity.
- Teach parents about need for eye prophylaxis. Educate them regarding side effects and signs that need to be reported to the healthcare provider.

Hepatitis B Vaccine (Engerix-B, Recombivax HB)

Overview of Neonatal Action

Recombinant hepatitis B vaccine is used as a prophylactic treatment against all subtypes of hepatitis B virus. It provides passive immunization for newborns of HBsAg-negative and HBsAg-positive mothers. Hepatitis B can be transmitted across the placenta, but most newborns are infected during birth.

The vaccine is produced from baker's yeast and plasmid containing the HBsAg gene.

Hepatitis B (thimerosal free) vaccine contains more than 95% HBsAg protein and is an inactivated (noninfective) product. Universal immunization is recommended.

Infants of HBsAg-positive mothers should concurrently receive 0.5 mL of hepatitis B immunoglobulin (HBIG) prophylaxis at separate injection sites (AAP & ACOG, 2007; Wilson, Shannon, & Shields, 2009).

Pregnancy Risk Category: C

Route, Dosage, Frequency

The first dose of 0.5 mL (10 mcg) is given intramuscularly into the anterolateral thigh within 12 hours of birth for infants born to HBsAg-positive mothers. The second dose of vaccine is given at least 1 month after the first dose and followed by a final dose at least 4 months after the first dose and at least 3 months after the second dose, but not before 6 months of age.

Infants born to HBsAg-negative mothers receive their first dose of vaccine at birth, the second dose at 1 to 2 months, and the third dose at 6 to 18 months (AAP & ACOG, 2007).

Infants whose mother's HBsAg status is unknown should receive the same doses of vaccine as infants born to HBsAg-positive mothers.

Neonatal Side Effects

The only common side effect is soreness at the injection site. Occasionally, there is erythema, swelling, warmth, and induration at the injection site, irritability, or a low-grade fever (37.7°C [99.8°F]).

Nursing Considerations

Delay administration during active infection, as the vaccine will not prevent infection during its incubation period.

- The vaccine should be used as supplied. Do not dilute. Shake well.
- Do not inject intravenously or interdermally.
- Monitor for adverse reactions. Monitor temperature closely.
- Have epinephrine available to treat possible allergic reactions.
- Responsiveness to the vaccine is age dependent. Preterm infants weighing less than 1,000 g have lower seroconversion rates. Consider delaying the first dose until the infant is term postconceptual age (PCA) or use a four-dose schedule.

MAGNESIUM SULFATE

Pregnancy Risk Category: B

Overview of Obstetric Action

Magnesium sulfate acts as a CNS depressant by decreasing the quantity of acetylcholine released by motor nerve impulses and thereby blocking neuromuscular transmission. This action reduces the possibility of convulsion, which is why magnesium sulfate is used in the treatment of preeclampsia. Because magnesium sulfate secondarily relaxes smooth muscle, it may decrease the blood pressure, although it is not considered an antihypertensive. Magnesium sulfate may also decrease the frequency and intensity of uterine contractions; as a result it is also used as a tocolytic in the treatment of preterm labor.

Route, Dosage, Frequency

Magnesium sulfate is generally given intravenously to control dosage more accurately and prevent overdosage. The intravenous route allows for immediate onset of action. It must be given by infusion pump for accurate dosage.

For Treatment of Preterm Labor

Loading dose: 4 to 8 g magnesium sulfate in a 10% to 20% solution administered over a 20- to 60-minute period.

Maintenance dose: 2 to 4 g/hr via infusion pump (Carey & Gibbs, 2008).

For Treatment of Preeclampsia

Loading dose: 4 to 6 g magnesium sulfate administered over a 20- to 30-minute period.

Maintenance dose: 2 to 3 g/hr via infusion pump (Habli & Sibai, 2008).

Note: Magnesium sulfate is excreted via the kidneys. Because women in preterm labor typically have normal renal function, they generally require higher levels of magnesium to achieve a therapeutic range than women who have preeclampsia and may have compromised renal function. Maintenance dose may need to be adjusted based on serum magnesium levels.

Maternal Contraindications

Diagnosed maternal myasthenia gravis is the only absolute contraindication to the administration of magnesium sulfate. A history of myocardial damage or heart block is a relative contraindication to use of the drug because of the effects on nerve transmission and muscle contractility. Extreme care is necessary in administration to women with impaired renal function because the drug is eliminated by the kidneys, and toxic magnesium levels may develop quickly.

Maternal Side Effects

Most maternal side effects are dose related. Lethargy and weakness related to neuromuscular blockade are common. Sweating, a feeling of warmth, flushing, and nasal congestion may be related to peripheral vasodilation. Other common side effects include nausea and vomiting, constipation, visual blurring, headache, and slurred speech. Signs of developing toxicity include depression or absence of reflexes, oliguria, confusion, respiratory depression, circulatory collapse, and respiratory paralysis. Rapid administration of large doses may cause cardiac arrest. If any of these occur, the drip should be stopped immediately.

Effects on Fetus/Newborn

The drug readily crosses the placenta. Some authorities suggest that transient decrease in FHR variability may occur; others report that no change occurred. In general, magnesium sulfate therapy does not pose a risk to the fetus. Occasionally, the newborn may demonstrate neurologic depression or respiratory depression, loss of reflexes, and muscle weakness. Ill effects in the newborn may actually be related to fetal growth retardation, prematurity, or perinatal asphyxia.

Nursing Considerations

- Monitor the blood pressure every 10 to 15 minutes during administration.
- Monitor maternal serum magnesium levels as ordered (usually every 6 to 8 hours). Therapeutic levels are in the range of 4 to 8 mg/dL. Reflexes often disappear at serum magnesium levels of 9 to 13 mg/dL; respiratory depression occurs at levels of 14 mg/dL;

cardiac arrest occurs at levels above 30 mg/L (Rideout, 2005).

- Monitor respirations closely. If the rate is less than 12/minute, magnesium toxicity may be developing, and further assessments are indicated. Many protocols require stopping the medication if the respiratory rate falls below 12/minute.

- Assess knee jerk (patellar tendon reflex) for evidence of diminished or absent reflexes. Loss of reflexes is often the first sign of developing toxicity. Also note marked lethargy or decreased level of consciousness and hypotension.

- Determine urinary output. Output less than 30 mL/hr may result in the accumulation of toxic levels of magnesium.

- If the respirations or urinary output fall below specified levels or if the reflexes are diminished or absent, no further magnesium should be administered until these factors return to normal.

- The antagonist of magnesium sulfate is calcium. Consequently, an ampule of calcium gluconate should be available at the bedside. The usual dose is 1 g given IV over a period of about 3 minutes.

- Monitor fetal heart tones continuously with IV administration.

- Continue magnesium sulfate infusion for approximately 24 hours after birth as prophylaxis against postpartum seizures if given for preeclampsia.

- If the mother has received magnesium sulfate close to birth, the newborn should be closely observed for signs of magnesium toxicity for 24 to 48 hours.

- The antidote for magnesium sulfate is calcium gluconate. Calcium gluconate should always be on hand in case the magnesium levels get too high.

Note: Protocols for magnesium sulfate administration may vary somewhat according to agency policy. Consequently, individuals are referred to their own agency protocols for specific guidelines.

Methylergonovine Maleate (Methergine)

Overview of Action

Methylergonovine maleate (Methergine) is an ergot alkaloid that stimulates smooth muscle tissue. Because the smooth muscle of the uterus is especially sensitive to this drug, it is used postpartally to stimulate the uterus to contract in order to decrease blood loss by clamping off uterine blood vessels and to promote the involution process. In addition, the drug has a vasoconstrictive effect on all blood vessels, especially the larger arteries. This may result in hypertension, particularly in a woman whose blood pressure is already elevated.

Route, Dosage, and Frequency

Methergine has a rapid onset of action and may be given orally or intramuscularly.

Usual IM dose: 0.2 mg following expulsion of the placenta. The dose may be repeated every 2 to 4 hours if necessary.

Usual oral dose: 0.2 mg every 4 hours (six doses).

Maternal Contraindications

Pregnancy, hepatic or renal disease, cardiac disease, hypertension, or preeclampsia contraindicate this drug's use. Methylergonovine maleate must be used with caution during lactation (Wilson, Shannon, & Shields, 2009).

Maternal Side Effects

Hypertension, nausea, vomiting, headache, bradycardia, dizziness, tinnitus, abdominal cramps, palpitations, dyspnea, chest pain, and allergic reactions may be noted.

Effects on Fetus or Newborn

Because Methergine has a long duration (3 hours [Wilson et al., 2009]) and action and can thus produce tetanic contractions, it *should never be used during pregnancy or in labor*, when it may result in a sustained uterine contraction that may cause amniotic fluid embolism (increased pressure in uterus may allow entry of amniotic fluid under the edge of the placenta and thus entry into the maternal venous system), uterine rupture, cervical and perineal lacerations (resulting from tetanic contractions and rapid birth of the baby), and hypoxia and intracranial hemorrhage in the baby (because of tetanic contractions, which severely decrease the maternal-placental-fetal blood flow, or uterine rupture, which causes cessation of blood flow to the unborn baby) (Wilson et al., 2009).

Nursing Considerations

- Monitor fundal height and consistency and the amount and character of the lochia.
- Assess the blood pressure before and routinely throughout drug administration.
- Observe for adverse effects or symptoms of ergot toxicity (ergotism), such as nausea and vomiting, headache, muscle pain, cold or numb fingers and toes, chest pain, and general weakness (Wilson et al., 2009).
- Provide client and family teaching regarding importance of not smoking during Methergine administration (nicotine from cigarettes leads to constricted vessels and may lead to hypertension) and signs of toxicity.

NALBUPHINE HYDROCHLORIDE (NUBAIN)

Overview of Action

Nubain is a synthetic opioid analgesic with agonist and weak antagonist properties. Analgesic properties are equal to those produced by morphine. Nubain's potency is three to four times greater than that of pentazocine. The incidence of respiratory depression that occurs is equivalent to that of morphine.

Dosage Route

Nubain is indicated for moderate to severe pain. Adults: 10 to 20 mg every 3 to 6 hours PRN subcutaneous/IM/IV.

Maternal Contraindications

Hypersensitivity or allergy to nalbuphine hydrochloride, respiratory depression, acute asthma attack, bradycardia, inflammatory bowel disease, and substance abuse.

Maternal Side Effects

Abdominal pain with cramps, allergic dermatitis, allergic reactions, angioedema, anorexia, atelectasis, biliary spasm, blurred vision, bradycardia, bronchial asthma, bronchospastic pulmonary disease, depression, diplopia, dizziness, drowsiness, dysgeusia, dyspnea, fainting, false sense of well-being, flushing, gastrointestinal irritation, general weakness, hallucinations, headache disorder, hypertension, hypotension, impaired cognition, insomnia, laryngeal edema, laryngismus, malaise, nausea, nervousness, nightmares, oliguria, pruritus of skin, pulse changes, respiratory depression, skin rash, tachyarrhythmia, ureteral spasm, urticaria, vertigo, visual changes, vomiting, xerostomia.

Nursing Considerations

- Assess client's allergy, sensitivity, or dependence to opioids on admission.
- Inform woman of potential side effects.
- Monitor and evaluate analgesic effect. Ask client about comfort level and notify analgesia provider of inadequate pain relief.
- Observe for symptoms of hypersensitivity: pruritus, urticaria, and/or burning sensation.
- May produce an allergic response in clients with sulfite sensitivity.
- If allergic reaction (urticaria, edema, or respiratory difficulties) occurs, administer naloxone or diphenhydramine per physician order.
- Assess respiratory rate before administration. Notify healthcare provider if respirations are less than 12 per minute.
- Monitor urinary output and assess bladder for distention. Assist client to void.

- Maintain bedrest or assist client with ambulation after administration.
- Counsel client that use with alcohol or other central nervous system depressants may increase medication effects.
- Prolonged use with abrupt discontinuation can result in symptoms consistent with opioid withdrawal in both the mother and infant.

Naloxone Hydrochloride (Narcan)

Overview of Neonatal Action

Naloxone hydrochloride (Narcan) is used to reverse respiratory depression caused by acute narcotic toxicity when the mother received a narcotic within 4 hours of birth. It displaces morphine-like drugs from receptor sites on the neurons; therefore the narcotics can no longer exert their depressive effects. It is essentially a pure opioid antagonist. Naloxone reverses narcotic-induced respiratory depression, analgesia, sedation, hypotension, and pupillary constriction.

Route, Dosage, Frequency

Intravenous dose is 0.1 mg/kg (0.25 mL/kg of 0.4 mg/mL concentration) at birth, including for premature infants. This drug is usually given through the umbilical vein or endotracheal tube (ET), although naloxone can be given intramuscularly (delays onset of action) if adequate perfusion exists. For IV push, infuse over at least 1 minute; for ET administration dilute in 1 to 2 milliliters of normal saline (NS).

Reversal of drug depression occurs within 1 to 2 minutes after IV administration and within 15 minutes of IM administration. The duration of action is variable (minutes to hours) and depends on the amount of the drug present and the rate of excretion. Duration of narcotic action often exceeds that of the naloxone. The dose may be repeated in 3 to 5 minutes. If there is no improvement after two or three doses, discontinue naloxone administration. If the initial reversal occurs, repeat the dose as needed (Young & Mangum, 2007).

Neonatal Contraindications

Naloxone should not be administered to infants of mothers who chronically use narcotics or those on methadone maintenance because it may precipitate acute withdrawal syndrome (increased heart rate and blood pressure, vomiting, seizures, tremors).

Respiratory depression may result from nonmorphine drugs, such as sedatives, hypnotics, anesthetics, or other nonnarcotic central nervous system (CNS) depressants.

Neonatal Side Effects

Excessive doses may result in irritability, increased crying, and possible prolongation of partial thromboplastin time (PTT).

Tachycardia may occur.

Nursing Considerations

- Monitor respirations—rate and depth—closely for improved respiratory effort.
- Assess for return of respiratory depression when naloxone effects wear off and effects of longer-acting narcotics reappear.
- Assess continued respiratory depression after positive-pressure ventilation has restored normal heart rate and color.
- Have resuscitative equipment, O_2, and ventilatory equipment available.
- Note that naloxone is incompatible with alkaline solutions such as sodium bicarbonate.
- Store at room temperature and protect from light.
- Remember that naloxone is compatible with heparin.

Oxytocin (Pitocin)

Overview of Obstetric Action

Oxytocin (Pitocin) exerts a selective stimulatory effect on the smooth muscle of the uterus and blood vessels. Oxytocin affects the myometrial cells of the uterus by increasing the excitability of the muscle cell, increasing the strength of the muscle contraction, and supporting propagation of the contraction (movement of the contraction from one myometrial cell to the next). Its effect on the uterine contraction depends on the dosage used and on the excitability of the myometrial cells. During the first half of gestation, there is little excitability of the myometrium, and the uterus is fairly resistant to the effects of oxytocin. However, from midgestation on, the uterus responds increasingly to exogenous intravenous oxytocin. Cautious use of diluted oxytocin administered intravenously at term results in a slow rise of uterine activity.

The circulatory half-life of oxytocin is 3 to 5 minutes. It takes approximately 40 minutes for a particular dose of oxytocin to reach a steady-state plasma concentration (Wilson et al., 2006).

The effects of oxytocin on the cardiovascular system can be pronounced. Blood pressure initially may decrease, but after prolonged administration increases by 30% above the baseline. Cardiac output and stroke volume increase. With doses of 20 milliunits/min or above, oxytocin exerts an antidiuretic effect decreasing free water exchange in the kidney and markedly decreasing urine output.

Oxytocin is used to induce labor at term and to augment uterine contractions in the first and second stages of labor. Oxytocin may also be used immediately after birth to stimulate uterine contraction and thereby control uterine atony.

Route, Dosage, Frequency

For induction of labor: Add 10 units of Pitocin (1 mL) to 1,000 mL of intravenous solution. (The resulting concentration is 10 mU oxytocin per 1 mL of intravenous fluid.) Using an infusion pump, administer IV, starting at 0.5–1 milliunit/min and increase by 1–2 milliunits/min every 40–60 minutes. Alternatively, start at 1–2 milliunits/min and increase by 1 milliunit/min every 15 minutes until a good contraction pattern (every 2–3 minutes and lasting 40–60 seconds) is achieved.

Maternal Contraindications

- Severe preeclampsia-eclampsia
- Predisposition to uterine rupture (in nullipara over 35 years of age, multigravida 4 or more, overdistention of the uterus, previous major surgery of the cervix or uterus)
- Cephalopelvic disproportion
- Malpresentation or malposition of the fetus, cord prolapse
- Preterm infant
- Rigid, unripe cervix; total placenta previa
- Presence of nonreassuring fetal status

Maternal Side Effects

Hyperstimulation of the uterus results in hypercontractility, which in turn may cause the following:

- Abruptio placentae
- Impaired uterine blood flow, leading to fetal hypoxia
- Rapid labor, leading to cervical lacerations
- Rapid labor and birth, leading to lacerations of cervix, vagina, or perineum, uterine atony; fetal trauma
- Uterine rupture
- Water intoxication (nausea, vomiting, hypotension, tachycardia, cardiac arrhythmia) if oxytocin is given in electrolyte-free solution or at a rate exceeding 20 milliunits/min; hypotension with rapid IV bolus administration postpartum

Effect on Fetus-Newborn

- Fetal effects are primarily associated with the presence of hypercontractility of the maternal uterus.

Hypercontractility decreases the oxygen supply to the fetus, which is reflected by irregularities or decrease in fetal heart rate (FHR)

- Hyperbilirubinemia (Wilson et al., 2006)
- Trauma from rapid birth

Nursing Considerations

- Explain induction or augmentation procedure to client.
- Apply fetal monitor, and obtain 15- to 20-minute tracing and nonstress test (NST) to assess FHR before starting IV oxytocin.
- For induction or augmentation of labor, start with primary IV, and piggyback secondary IV with oxytocin and infusion pump.
- Ensure continuous monitoring of the fetus and uterine contractions.
- The maximum rate is 40 milliunits/min (Blackburn, 2007). Not all protocols recommend a maximum dose. When indicated, the maximum dose is generally between 16 and 40 milliunits/min. Decrease oxytocin by similar increments once labor has progressed to 5–6 cm dilatation. Protocols may vary from one agency to another.

0.5 milliunit/min = 3 mL/hr

1.0 milliunit/min = 6 mL/hr

1.5 milliunit/min = 9 mL/hr

2 milliunit/min = 12 mL/hr

4 milliunit/min = 24 mL/hr

6 milliunit/min = 36 mL/hr

8 milliunit/min = 48 mL/hr

10 milliunit/min = 60 mL/hr

12 milliunit/min = 72 mL/hr

15 milliunit/min = 90 mL/hr

18 milliunit/min = 108 mL/hr

20 milliunit/min = 120 mL/hr

- Assess FHR, maternal blood pressure, pulse, frequency and duration of uterine contractions, and uterine resting tone before each increase in the oxytocin infusion rate.
- Record all assessments and IV rate on monitor strip and on client's chart.
- Record oxytocin infusion rate in milliunits/min and mL/hr (e.g., 0.5 milliunits/min [3 mL/hr]).
- Record on monitor strip all client activities (such as change of position, vomiting), procedures done (amniotomy, sterile vaginal examination), and administration of analgesic agents to allow for interpretation and evaluation of tracing.
- Assess cervical dilatation as needed.
- Apply nursing comfort measures.
- Discontinue IV oxytocin infusion and infuse primary solution when (1) nonreassuring fetal status is noted (bradycardia, late or variable decelerations); (2) uterine contractions are more frequent than every 2 minutes; (3) duration of contractions exceeds more than 60 seconds; or (4) insufficient relaxation of the uterus between contractions or a steady increase in resting tone is noted (Blackburn, 2007). In addition to discontinuing IV oxytocin infusion, turn client to side, and if nonreassuring fetal status is present, administer oxygen by tight face mask at 7–10 L/min; notify physician.
- Maintain intake and output record.

For Augmentation of Labor

Prepare and administer IV Pitocin as for labor induction. Increase rate until labor contractions are of good quality. The flow rate is gradually increased at no less than every 30 minutes to a maximum of 10 milliunits/min (Blackburn, 2007). In some settings or in a situation when limited fluids may be administered, a more concentrated solution may be used. When 10 units Pitocin are added to 500-mL IV solution, the resulting concentration is 1 milliunit/min = 3 mL/hr. If 10 units Pitocin are added to 250-mL IV solution, the concentration is 1 milliunit/min = 1.5 mL/hr.

For Administration After Expulsion of Placenta

- One dose of 10 units of Pitocin (1 mL) is given intramuscularly or added to IV fluids for continuous infusion.

- Assess FHR, maternal blood pressure, pulse, frequency and duration of uterine contractions, and uterine resting tone before each increase in oxytocin infusion rate.

- Record all assessments and IV rate on monitor strip and on client's chart. Record oxytocin infusion rate in milliunits/min and mL/hr (e.g., 0.5 milliunits/min [3 mL/hr]).

- Record on monitor strip all client activities (such as change of position, vomiting), procedures done (amniotomy, sterile vaginal examination), and administration of analgesic agents to allow for interpretation and evaluation of tracing.

- Assess cervical dilatation as needed.

- Apply nursing comfort measures.

- Discontinue IV oxytocin infusion and infuse primary solution when (1) nonreassuring fetal status is noted (tachycardia or bradycardia, late or variable decelerations), (2) uterine contractions are more frequent than every 2 minutes, (3) duration of contractions exceeds 60 seconds, or (4) insufficient relaxation of the uterus between contractions or a steady increase in resting tone is noted (Blackburn, 2007). In addition to discontinuing IV oxytocin infusion, turn client to side, and if nonreassuring fetal status is present, administer oxygen by tight face mask at 7–10 L/min; notify physician.

- Maintain intake and output record. Assess intake and output every hour.

Postpartum Epidural Morphine

Overview of Obstetric Action

Epidural morphine is used to provide relief of pain associated with cesarean birth, extensive episiotomies (mediolaterals), or third- and fourth-degree lacerations. Epidural morphine pain relief results directly from its effect on the opiate receptors in the spinal cord (it depresses pain impulse transmission). Morphine binds opiate receptors, thereby altering both the perception of and emotional response to pain. Women experience little or no discomfort or pain during recovery and for up to 24 hours afterward. There is no motor or sympathetic block or associated hypotension. Onset of analgesia is slower, but duration is longer.

Route, Dosage, and Frequency

Morphine (5 to 7.5 mg) is injected through a catheter into the epidural space, providing pain relief for about 24 hours (Wilson et al., 2009).

Maternal Contraindications

Allergy to morphine, narcotic addiction, chronic debilitating respiratory disease, infection at the injection site, or administration of parenteral corticosteroids in past 14 days (Wilson et al., 2009).

Maternal Side Effects

Late-onset respiratory depression (rare but may occur 8 to 12 hours after administration), nausea and vomiting (occurring between 4 and 7 hours after injection), itching (begins within 3 hours and lasts up to 10 hours), urinary retention, and rarely somnolence. Side effects can be managed with naloxone.

Neonatal Effects

No adverse effects because medication is injected after the birth of the baby.

Nursing Considerations

- Obtain history: sensitivity (allergy) to morphine, presence of any contraindications (Wilson et al., 2009).
- Assess orientation, reflexes, skin color, texture, breath sounds, presence of lesions or infection over area of lumbar spine, voiding pattern, urinary output within normal limits (Wilson et al., 2009).
- Monitor and evaluate analgesic effect. Ask client about comfort level and notify anesthesiologist of inadequate pain relief.
- Check catheter for obvious knots, breaks, and leakage at insertion site and catheter hub.
- Assess for pruritus (scratching and rubbing, especially around face and neck).
- Administer comfort measures for narcotic-induced pruritus, such as lotion, backrubs, cool/warm packs, or diversional activities. If the itching can be tolerated, naloxone should be avoided, especially because it counteracts the pain relief.
- If allergic reaction (urticaria, edema, or respiratory difficulties) occurs, administer naloxone or diphenhydramine per physician order.
- Provide comfort measures for nausea/vomiting, such as frequent oral hygiene or gradual increase of activity; administer naloxone, trimethobenzamide (Tigan), or metoclopramide HCl per physician order.
- Assess postural blood pressure and heart rate before ambulation.
- Assist client with her first ambulation and then as needed.
- Assess respiratory function every hour for 24 hours, then q2–8 hr as needed. Also assess level of consciousness and mucous membrane color. May need to monitor client via apnea monitor for 24 hours.
- Monitor urinary output and assess bladder for distention. Assist client to void.

Vitamin K₁ Phytonadione (AquaMEPHYTON)

Overview of Neonatal Action

Phytonadione is used in prophylaxis and treatment of vitamin K deficiency bleeding (VKDB), formerly known as hemorrhagic disease of the newborn. It promotes liver formation of the clotting factors II, VII, IX, and X. At birth, the newborn does not have the bacteria in the colon that are necessary for synthesizing fat-soluble vitamin K_1. Therefore, the newborn may have decreased levels of prothrombin during the first 5 to 8 days of life, reflected by a prolongation of prothrombin time.

Pregnancy Risk Category: C

Route, Dosage, Frequency

Intramuscular injection is given in the vastus lateralis thigh muscle. A one-time-only prophylactic dose of 0.5 to 1 mg is given intramuscularly within 1 hour of birth or may be delayed until after the first breast-feeding in the delivery/birthing area (AAP & ACOG, 2007, Wilson, Shannon, & Shields, 2009).

If the mother received anticoagulants during pregnancy, an additional dose may be ordered by the physician and is given 6 to 8 hours after the first injection. IM concentration: 1 mg/0.5 mL (neonatal strength); can use 10 mg/mL concentration to minimize volume injected.

Neonatal Side Effects

Pain and edema may occur at the injection site. Allergic reactions, such as rash and urticaria, may also occur.

Nursing Considerations

- Protect drug from light.
- Give vitamin K_1 before circumcision procedure.
- Observe for signs of local inflammation.

- Observe for bleeding (usually occurs on second or third day). Bleeding may be seen as generalized ecchymoses or bleeding from umbilical cord, circumcision site, nose, or gastrointestinal tract. Results of serial prothrombin time (PT) and international normalized ratio (INR) should be assessed.
- Observe for jaundice and kernicterus, especially in preterm infants.

Procedures

Administration of Rh Immune Globulin (RhoGAM, HypRho-D)

Preparation

1. Confirm that Rh immune globulin is indicated by checking the woman's prenatal or intrapartal record to verify that she is Rh negative. Then confirm that sensitization has not occurred—maternal indirect Coombs' negative. Postpartally, confirm that the baby is Rh positive but not sensitized (direct Coombs' negative) and that the mother's indirect Coombs' is negative. Rh immune globulin is *not* indicated if the infant is Rh negative, too.

   Rationale: Rh immune globulin is only indicated for Rh-negative, unsensitized women.

2. Confirm that the woman does not have a history of allergies to immune globulin preparations by checking entries on medication allergies in her chart and by asking her whether she has ever had any allergic reactions to medications, globulins, or blood products.

   Rationale: Rh immune globulin is made from the plasma portion of blood. Allergic reactions are possible.

3. Explain purpose and procedure. Have consent form signed if required by agency policy.

Rationale: Many agencies require separate consent for the administration of Rh immune globulin because it is a blood product.

Rationale: The woman should clearly understand the purpose of the Rh immune globulin, its rationale, the administration procedure, and any related risks. Generally the primary side effects are redness and tenderness at the injection site and allergic responses.

Equipment and Supplies

- Rh immune globulin, which is obtained from the blood bank or pharmacy according to agency protocol. Lot numbers for the drug and the crossmatch should be the same.
- Syringe and IM needle.

Procedure

1. Confirm the woman's identity and administer one vial of 300-mcg Rh immune globulin IM into the deltoid muscle.

2. An immune globulin microdose is used after miscarriage, elective abortion, ectopic pregnancy, or molar pregnancy occurring within the first 12 weeks' gestation. Antepartally, the Rh immune globulin is generally given within 3 hours but not longer than 72 hours of the event.

3. If a larger bleed is suspected at birth (as in cases of severe abruptio placentae), additional doses may be administered at one time using multiple sites or at regular intervals as long as all doses are given within 72 hours of childbirth.

Rationale: The normal 300-mcg dose provides passive immunity following exposure of up to 15 mL of transfused RBCs or 30 mL of fetal blood.

4. Provide opportunities for the woman to ask questions and express concerns.

Rationale: Many women, especially primigravidas, are not aware of the risks for an Rh-positive fetus of a sensitized Rh-negative mother. They need to understand the importance of receiving

Rh immune globulin for each pregnancy to ensure continued protection.

5. Chart according to agency policy. Most agencies chart lot number, route, dose, and client education.

Assessing Deep Tendon Reflexes and Clonus

Preparation

1. Explain the procedure, indications for its use, and information that will be obtained.
2. Most nurses check the patellar reflex and one other, such as the biceps, triceps, or brachioradialis.

   Rationale: DTRs are assessed to gain information about CNS irritability secondary to preeclampsia and to assess the effects of magnesium sulfate if the woman is receiving it.

Equipment and Supplies

- Percussion hammer

Procedure

1. Elicit reflexes.
   - Patellar reflex. Position the woman with her legs hanging over the edge of the bed (feet should not be touching the floor) (see Figure 1). Briskly strike the patellar tendon, which is located just below the patella. Normal response is extension or a thrusting forward of the foot.

     Rationale: In an inpatient setting the patellar reflex is often assessed while the woman lies supine. Flex her knees slightly and support them.
   - Biceps reflex. Flex the woman's arm 45 degrees at the elbow and place your thumb on the biceps tendon. Allow your fingers to hold the biceps muscle. Strike your thumb in a slightly downward motion and assess the response. Normal response is flexion of the arm.

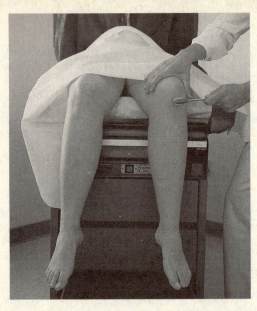

Figure 1 ■ Correct position for eliciting patellar reflex: sitting.

- Triceps reflex. Flex the woman's arm up to 90 degrees and allow her hand to hang against the side of her body. Using the percussion hammer, strike the triceps tendon just above the elbow. Normal response is contraction of the muscle, which causes extension of the arm.
- Brachioradialis reflex. Flex the woman's arm slightly and lay it on your forearm with her hand slightly pronated. Using the percussion hammer, strike the brachioradialis tendon, which is found about 1 to 2 inches above the wrist. Normal response is pronation of the forearm and flexion of the elbow.

  Rationale: The correct position causes the muscle to be slightly stretched. Then when the tendon is stretched, with a tap the muscle should contract. Correct positioning and technique are essential to elicit the reflex.

2. Grade reflexes. Reflexes are graded on a scale of 0 to 4+, as follows:

   4+ Hyperactive; very brisk, jerky, or clonic response; abnormal

   3+ Brisker than average; may not be abnormal

   2+ Average response; normal

   1+ Diminished response; low normal

   0 No response; abnormal

   Rationale: Normally reflexes are 1+ or 2+. With CNS irritation, hyperreflexia may be present; with high magnesium levels, reflexes may be diminished or absent.

3. Assess for clonus. With the woman's knee flexed and the leg supported, vigorously dorsiflex the foot, maintain the dorsiflexion momentarily, and then release (Figure 2). With a normal response, the

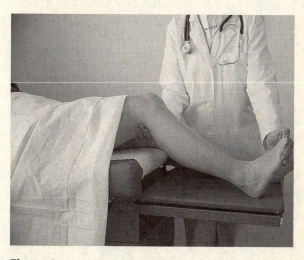

Figure 2 ■ To elicit clonus, sharply dorsiflex the foot.

foot returns to its normal position of plantar flexion. Clonus is present if the foot "jerks" or taps against the examiner's hand. If so, record the number of taps or beats of clonus.

Rationale: Clonus occurs with more pronounced hyperreflexia and indicates CNS irritability.

4. Report and record findings. For example: DTRs 2+, no clonus or DTRs 4+, 2 beats clonus.

Assessing the Status of the Uterine Fundus after Birth

Preparation

1. Explain the procedure, the information it provides, and what it might feel like.

2. Ask the woman to void.

   Rationale: A full bladder can cause uterine atony.

3. Have the woman lie flat in bed with her head on a pillow. If the procedure is uncomfortable, she may find that it helps to flex her legs.

   Rationale: The supine position prevents falsely high assessment of fundal height. Flexing the legs relaxes the abdominal muscles.

Equipment and Supplies

Clinical Tip Gloves may be put on before assessing the abdomen and fundus or when you are ready to assess the perineum and lochia.

• A clean perineal pad (see Clinical Skill: Evaluating Lochia)

Procedure

1. Gently place one hand on the lower segment of the uterus. Using the side of the other hand, palpate the abdomen until you locate the top of the fundus.

Rationale: One hand stabilizes the uterus while the other hand locates the top of the fundus. (Support of the uterus prevents stretching of the ligaments that support the uterus.)

2. Determine whether the fundus is firm. If it is, it will feel like a hard, round object (similar to a grapefruit) in the abdomen. If it is not firm, massage the abdomen lightly until the fundus is firm.

   Rationale: A firm fundus indicates that the uterine muscles are contracted and bleeding will not occur.

3. Measure the top of the fundus in finger breadths above, below, or at the fundus. See Figure 3.

   Rationale: Fundal height gives information about the progress of involution.

4. Determine the position of the fundus in relation to the midline of the body. If it is not in the midline, locate it and then evaluate the bladder for distention.

   Rationale: The fundus may deviate from the midline when the bladder is full because the enlarged bladder pushes the uterus aside.

5. If the bladder is distended, use nursing measures to help the woman void. If she is not able to void after

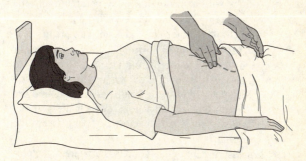

Figure 3 ■ Measurement of descent of fundus for the woman with vaginal birth. The fundus is located two finger breadths below the umbilicus.

a specified period of time, catheterization may be necessary.

6. Measure urine output for the next few hours until normal elimination is established.

   Rationale: During the postpartum as diuresis occurs; the bladder may fill far more rapidly than normal, putting the woman at risk for uterine atony and hemorrhage. (Diminished tone of the uterus may cause loss of the urge to void.)

7. Assess the lochia (see Clinical Skill: Evaluating Lochia).

8. During the first few hours postpartum, if the fundus becomes boggy frequently or is located high above the umbilicus and the woman's bladder is empty, the uterine cavity may be filled with clots of blood. In this case, do the following:

   Rationale: If the woman's uterus is filled with blood, it acts as an irritant and the uterus will not remain contracted. When the muscle fibers relax, bleeding results, further aggravating the problem. Pushing on a uterus that is not firm is dangerous because it is possible to cause the uterus to invert, which is a true emergency.

   - Release the front of the perineal pad and lay it back so that you can see the perineum and the pad laying between the woman's legs.
   - Massage the uterine fundus until it is firm.
   - Keep one hand in position stabilizing the lower portion of the uterus. With the hand you used to massage the fundus, put steady pressure on the top of the now-firm fundus and see if you are able to express any clots. (Watch the pad between her legs for clots to pass from the vagina.)

9. If measurement of the blood loss is needed, the perineal pads and Chux can be weighed (see Clinical Skill: Evaluating Lochia).

10. Provide the woman with a clean perineal pad.

11. Record findings. Fundal height is recorded in finger breadths (e.g., "2 FB ↓ U" or "1 FB ↑ U"). If fundal massage was necessary, note that fact: "Uterus boggy → firm with light massage."
12. Communicate bogginess or heavy flow to primary provider.

ASSISTING DURING AMNIOCENTESIS

Preparation

- Explain the procedure, the indications for it, and reassure the woman.

    Rationale: Explanation of the procedure decreases anxiety.

- Determine whether an informed consent has been signed. If not, verify that the woman's doctor has explained the procedure and ask her to sign a consent form.

    Rationale: It is the physician's responsibility to obtain informed consent. The woman's signature indicates her awareness of risks and gives her consent to the procedure.

Equipment and Supplies

Prepare and arrange the following items so they are easily accessible:

- 22-gauge spinal needle with stylet
- 10 and 20 mL syringes
- 1% xylocaine
- Povidone–iodine (Betadine)
- Three 10-mL test tubes with tops (amber colored or covered with tape)

    Rationale: Amniotic fluid must be shielded from light to prevent breakdown of bilirubin.

Procedure: Sterile Gloves

1. Obtain baseline vital signs data on maternal BP, temperature, pulse, respirations, and FHR before

procedure begins; then monitor BP, pulse, respirations, and FHR every 15 minutes during procedure.

Rationale: Baseline information is essential to detect any changes in maternal or fetal status that might be related to the procedure.

2. Provide gel for the ultrasound and assist with the real-time ultrasound to assess needle insertion during the procedure as needed.

Rationale: Amniocentesis is usually performed laterally in the area of fetal small parts, where pockets of amniotic fluid are often seen. Real-time ultrasound will identify fetal parts and locate pockets of amniotic fluid.

3. Cleanse the woman's abdomen.

Rationale: Cleansing the woman's abdomen before needle insertion helps decrease the risk of infection.

4. The physician dons gloves, inserts the needle into the identified pocket of fluid, and withdraws a sample.

5. Obtain the test tubes from the physician.

6. Label the tubes with the women's correct identification and send to the lab with the appropriate lab slips.

7. Monitor the woman and reassess her vital signs.
   • Determine the woman's BP, pulse, respirations, and FHR.
   • Palpate the woman's fundus to assess for uterine contractions.
   • Monitor the woman with an external fetal monitor for 20 to 30 minutes after the amniocentesis.
   • Determine a treatment course to counteract any supine hypotension and to increase venous return and cardiac output.

Rationale: Monitoring maternal and fetal status postprocedure provides information about response to the procedure and helps detect any complications such as inadvertent fetal puncture.

8. Assess the woman's blood type and determine any need for Rh immune globulin.

   Rationale: Rh immune globulin is administered prophylactically following an amniocentesis to prevent Rh sensitization in an Rh-negative woman.

9. Administer Rh immune globulin if indicated.

10. Reassure the woman and provide self-care education.
    - Instruct the woman to report any of the following changes or symptoms to her primary caregiver:
      a. Unusual fetal hyperactivity or, conversely, any lack of movement
      b. Vaginal discharge—clear drainage or bleeding
      c. Uterine contractions or abdominal pain
      d. Fever or chills

    Rationale: The woman will know how to recognize changes or symptoms that warrant further evaluation.

11. Encourage the woman to engage in only light activity for 24 hours and to increase her fluid intake.

    Rationale: A decrease in maternal activity will decrease uterine irritability and increase uteroplacental circulation. Increased hydration will replace the amniotic fluid through the uteroplacental circulation. Provides a permanent record.

12. Complete the client record.
    - Record the type of procedure, the date and time, name of the physician who performed the procedure, and the disposition of the specimen.
    - Record the maternal–fetal response such as maternal vital signs, level of discomfort, FHR, and presence of contractions, bleeding, and fluid leakage, if occurred. Discharge instructions given should be documented.

AUSCULTATION OF FETAL HEART RATE

Preparation

1. Explain the procedure, the indications for it, and the information that will be obtained.
2. Uncover the woman's abdomen.

Equipment and Supplies

- Doppler device
- Ultrasonic gel

Procedure

1. To use the Doppler:
   - Place ultrasonic gel on the diaphragm of the Doppler. Gel is used to maintain contact with the maternal abdomen and enhances conduction of sound.
   - Place the Doppler diaphragm on the woman's abdomen halfway between the umbilicus and symphysis and in the midline. You are most likely to hear the FHR in this area. Listen carefully for the sound of the fetal heartbeat.
2. Check the woman's pulse against the fetal sounds you hear. If the rates are the same, reposition the Doppler and try again.

   Rationale: If the rates are the same, you are probably hearing the maternal pulse and not the FHR.
3. If the rates are not similar, count the FHR for 1 full minute. Note that the FHR has a double rhythm and only one sound is counted.
4. If you do not locate the FHR, move the Doppler laterally.
5. Auscultate the FHR between, during, and for 30 seconds following a uterine contraction (UC).

6. Frequency recommendations:
   - *Low-risk women:* Every 1 hour in the latent phase, every 30 minutes in the active phase, and every 15 minutes in the second stage.
   - *High-risk women:* Every 30 minutes in the latent phase, every 15 minutes in the active phase, and every 5 minutes in the second stage.

   Rationale: This evaluation provides the opportunity to assess the fetal status and response to labor.

7. Document FHR data (rate and rhythm), characteristics of uterine activity, and any actions taken as a result of the FHR.

Auscultation with the Fetoscope

The fetoscope is an older assessment tool; however, some clinicians prefer it because it is "natural" and does not rely on ultrasound.

To use the fetoscope:

- Place the fetoscope earpieces in your ears; use the handpiece to position the bell of the fetoscope on the mother's abdomen.
- Place the diaphragm halfway between the umbilicus and symphysis and in the midline. *You are most likely to hear the FHR in this area.*
- Without touching the fetoscope, listen carefully for the FHR.

ELECTRONIC FETAL MONITORING

Preparation

Explain the procedure, the indications for it, and the information that will be obtained.

Equipment and Supplies

- Monitor
- Two elastic monitor belts
- Tocodynamometer ("toco")

- Ultrasound transducer
- Ultrasound gel

Procedure

1. Turn on the monitor.
2. Place the two elastic belts around the woman's abdomen.
3. Place the "toco" over the uterine fundus off the midline on the area palpated to be most firm during contractions. Secure it with one of the elastic belts.

   Rationale: The uterine fundus is the area of greatest contractility.

4. Note the UC tracing. The resting tone tracing (that is, without a UC) should be recording on the 10- or 15-mm-Hg pressure line. Adjust the line to reflect that reading.

   Rationale: If the resting tone is set on the zero line, there often is a constant grinding noise.

5. Apply the ultrasonic gel to the diaphragm of the ultrasound transducer.

   Rationale: Ultrasonic gel is used to maintain contact with the maternal abdomen. The ultrasonic beam is directed toward the fetal heart.

6. Place the diaphragm on the maternal abdomen in the midline between the umbilicus and the symphysis pubis.

7. Listen for the FHR, which will have a whiplike sound. Move the diaphragm laterally if necessary to obtain a stronger sound.

8. When the FHR is located, attach the second elastic belt snugly to the transducer.

   Rationale: Firm contact is necessary to maintain a steady tracing.

9. Place the following information on the beginning of the fetal monitor paper: date, time, woman's name, gravida, para, membrane status, and name of physician or certified nurse-midwife.

10. Ongoing documentation should provide information about FHR, including baseline rate in beats per minute (bpm), long-term variability (LTV), short-term variability (STV), response to uterine contractions (accelerations or decelerations), procedures performed, changes in position and the like, as well as any therapy initiated.

Note: Each birthing unit may have specific guidelines about additional information to include. A full description of fetal monitoring analysis is beyond the scope of this text.

EVALUATING LOCHIA

Preparation

1. Explain why lochia occurs, why it is assessed, how it is assessed, and how it changes during the postpartum.

2. Ask the woman to void.

   Rationale: A full bladder can cause uterine atony and increase the amount of lochia.

3. Complete the assessment of uterine fundal height and firmness.

   Rationale: In almost all cases, fundal height and firmness are evaluated with an assessment of lochia. This practice provides a more thorough assessment.

4. If she has not already done so for the fundal assessment, ask the woman to flex her legs. Then ask her to spread her legs apart. Use the bed sheet as a drape to preserve her modesty.

   Rationale: This position allows you to see the perineum and the perineal pad more effectively.

Equipment and Supplies

Note: Gloves are put on before assessing the perineum and lochia.

• Gloves
• Clean perineal pad

Procedures: Clean Gloves

1. Don gloves.
2. Lower the perineal pad and observe the amount of lochia on the pad. Because women's pad-changing practices vary, ask her about the length of time the current pad has been in use, whether the amount is normal, and whether any clots were passed before this examination, such as during voiding.

   Rationale: During the first 1 to 3 days the woman's lochia should be rubra, which is dark red in color. A few small clots are normal and occur as a result of pooling of blood in the vagina when the woman is lying down. The passage of large clots is abnormal and the cause should be investigated immediately.

Clinical Tip If blood loss exceeds the guidelines given in this chapter, weigh the perineal pads and the Chux pads to estimate the blood loss more accurately. Typically, 1g = 1mL blood. Because blood can pool below the woman on the chux pad, the pads are included in your assessment.

---

3. If the woman reports heavy bleeding or clots, ask her to put on a clean perineal pad and then reassess the pad in 1 hour. Also ask her to call you before flushing any clots she passes into the toilet during voiding.
4. When the uterine fundus is firm and stabilized with the nondominant hand, press down on it with the dominant hand while watching to see if any clots are expelled. (See Clinical Skill: Assessing the Status of the Uterine Fundus after Birth, step 8.)
5. Determine the amount of lochia, using the following guide (see Figure 4):
   • Heavy amount—Perineal pad has a stain larger than 6 inches in length within 1 hour; 30 to 80 mL lochia.
   • Moderate amount—Perineal pad has a stain less than 6 inches in length within 1 hour; 25 to 50 mL lochia.

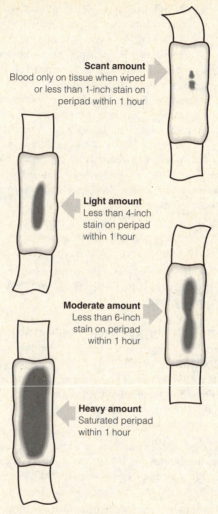

Scant amount
Blood only on tissue when wiped or less than 1-inch stain on peripad within 1 hour

Light amount
Less than 4-inch stain on peripad within 1 hour

Moderate amount
Less than 6-inch stain on peripad within 1 hour

Heavy amount
Saturated peripad within 1 hour

Figure 4 ■ Suggested guideline for assessing lochia volume.
Source: "A Standard for Assessing Lochia Volume," by H. Jacobson, May to June 1985, *Maternal-Child Nursing.*

- Small (light) amount—Perineal pad has a stain less than 4 inches in length after 1 hour; 10 to 25 mL lochia.
- Scant amount—Perineal pad has a stain less than 1 inch in length after 1 hour or lochia is only on tissue when the woman wipes.

  Rationale: Lochia should never exceed a moderate amount, such as 4 to 8 partially saturated perineal pads daily. Using a consistent standard for measuring lochia improves the accuracy of the information charted and conveyed to others.

6. In most cases, a woman is discharged while her lochia is still rubra. Provide her with information about lochia serosa and lochia alba.

   Rationale: Accurate discharge information enables the woman to assess herself more accurately and enables her to judge better when to contact her caregiver.

7. Record the findings specifically. For example, "Uterus firm, 1FB ↓ U, Lochia: moderate rubra, no clots passed."

Infant Receiving Phototherapy

Preparation

- Explain the purpose of phototherapy, the procedure itself (including the need to use eye patches), and possible side effects such as dehydration and skin breakdown from more frequent stooling.

- Note evidence of jaundice in skin, sclera, and mucous membranes (in infants with darkly pigmented skin). Be sure that recent serum bilirubin levels are available.

  Rationale: The decision to use phototherapy is based on a careful assessment of the newborn's condition over a period of time. The most recent results before starting therapy serve as a baseline to evaluate the effectiveness of therapy.

Equipment and Supplies
- Bank of phototherapy lights
- Eye patches
- Small scale to weigh diapers

Procedure
1. Obtain vital signs including axillary temperature.

   Rationale: Provides baseline data.

2. Remove all of the infant's clothing except the diaper.

   Rationale: Exposure of the newborn to high-intensity light (a bank of fluorescent light bulbs or bulbs in the blue-white spectrum) decreases serum bilirubin levels in the skin by aiding biliary excretion of unconjugated bilirubin. Because the tissue absorbs the light, best results are obtained when there is maximum skin surface exposure.

3. Apply eye coverings (eye patches or a bili mask) to the infant according to agency policy (see Figure 5).

   Rationale: Eye coverings are used because it is not known if phototherapy injures delicate eye structures, particularly the retina.

4. Place the infant in an open crib or incubator (more commonly used in preterm infants and infants who are sicker) about 45 to 50 cm below the bank of phototherapy lights.

   Rationale: The incubator helps the infant maintain his or her temperature while undressed.
   Reposition every 2 hours.

   Rationale: Repositioning exposes different areas of skin to the lights, prevents the development of pressure areas on the skin, and varies the stimulation the infant receives.

5. Monitor vital signs every 4 hours with axillary temperatures.

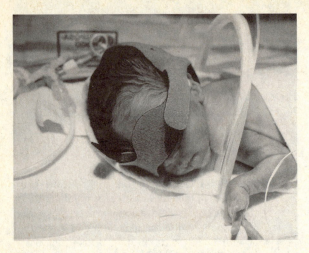

Figure 5 ▓ Infant receiving phototherapy. The phototherapy light is positioned over the incubator. Bilateral eye patches are always used during photo light therapy to protect the baby's eyes.

Source: Courtesy of Lisa Smith-Pedersen, RNC, MSN, NNP.

> **Rationale:** Temperature assessment is indicated to detect hypothermia or hyperthermia.
>
> Deviation in pulse and respirations may indicate developing complications.

6. Cluster care activities.

> **Rationale:** Care activities are clustered to help ensure that the newborn has maximum time under the lights.

7. Discontinue phototherapy and remove eye patches at least every 2 to 3 hours when feeding the infant and when the parents visit.

> **Rationale:** Eye patches are removed to assess for signs of complications such as excessive pressure, discharge, or conjunctivitis. Patches are also

removed to provide some social stimulation and to promote parental attachment.

8. Maintain adequate fluid intake. Evaluate need for IV fluids.

9. Monitor intake and output carefully. Weigh diapers before discarding. Record quantity and characteristics of each stool.

   Rationale: Infants undergoing phototherapy treatment have increased water loss through skin and loose stools. Loose stools and increased urine output are a result of bilirubin excretion. This increases their risk of dehydration.

10. Assess specific gravity with each voiding. Weigh newborn daily.

    Rationale: Specific gravity provides one measure of urine concentration. Highly concentrated urine is associated with a dehydrated state. Weight loss is also a sign of developing dehydration in the newborn.

11. Observe the infant for signs of perianal excoriation and institute therapy if it develops.

    Rationale: Perianal excoriation may develop because of the irritating effect of diarrhea stools.

12. Ensure that serum bilirubin levels are drawn regularly according to orders or agency policy. Turn the phototherapy lights off while the blood is drawn.

    Rationale: Serum bilirubin levels provide the most accurate indication of the effectiveness of phototherapy. They are generally drawn every 12 hours, but at least once daily. The phototherapy lights are turned off to ensure accurate serum bilirubin levels.

13. Examine the newborn's skin regularly for signs of developing pressure areas, bronzing, maculopapular rash, and changes in degree of jaundice.

Rationale: Pressure areas may develop if the infant lies in one position for an extended period. A benign, transient bronze discoloration of the skin may occur with phototherapy when the infant has elevated direct serum bilirubin levels or liver disease. A maculopapular rash is another transient side effect of phototherapy that develops occasionally.

14. Avoid using lotion or ointment on the exposed skin.

    Rationale: Lotion and ointments on a newborn receiving phototherapy may cause skin burns.

15. Provide parents with opportunities to hold the newborn and assist in the infant's care. Answer their questions accurately and keep them informed of developments or changes.

    Rationale: A sick infant is a source of great anxiety for parents. Information helps them deal with their anxiety. Moreover, they have a right to be kept well informed of their baby's status so that they are able to make informed decisions as needed.

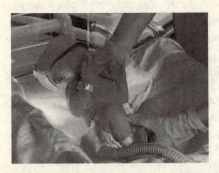

Figure 6 ■ Newborn on fiber-optic "Bili" mattress and under phototherapy lights. A combination of fiber-optic light source mattress and standard phototherapy light source above may also be used.

Note: The color is distorted because of the reflection of the bililight mattress.

16. May also provide phototherapy using lightweight, fiber-optic blankets ("bili blankets"). The baby is wrapped in the blanket, which is plugged into an outlet (see Figure 6).

Rationale: With fiber-optic blankets the newborn is readily accessible for care, feedings, and diaper changes. The baby does not get overheated, and fluid and weight loss are not complications of this system. The procedure seems less alarming to parents than standard phototherapy.

PERFORMING A HEEL STICK ON A NEWBORN

Preparation
- Explain to parents what will be done.
- Select a clear, previously unpunctured site.

    Rationale: The selection of a previously unpunctured site minimizes the risk of infection and excessive scar formation.

- The infant's lateral heel is the site of choice because it precludes damaging the posterior tibial nerve and artery, plantar artery, and the important longitudinally oriented fat pad of the heel, which in later years could impede walking (Figure 7). This is especially important for infants undergoing multiple heel stick procedures. Toes are acceptable sites if necessary.

Equipment and Supplies
- Microlancet (do not use a needle)

    Rationale: A needle may nick the periosteum.

- Alcohol swabs
- 2 × 2 sterile gauze squares
- Small bandage
- Transfer pipette or capillary tubes
- Glucose reagent strips and reflectance meters
- Gloves

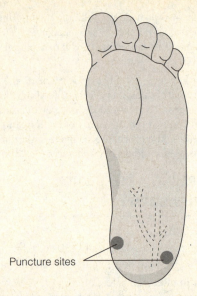

Puncture sites

Figure 7 ■ Potential sites for heel sticks. Avoid shaded areas to prevent injury to arteries and nerves in the foot.

Procedure

1. Apply gloves.

   Rationale: Gloves are used to implement standard precautions and prevent nosocomial infections.

2. May try warm wet wrap or specially designed chemical heat pad to warm the infant's heel for 5 to 10 seconds to facilitate blood flow.

Performing the Heel Stick

1. Grasp the infant's lower leg and foot so as to impede venous return slightly. This will facilitate extraction of the blood sample (Figure 8).

2. Clean the site by rubbing vigorously with 70% isopropyl alcohol swab.

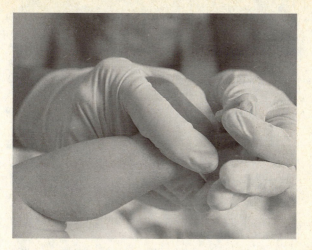

Figure 8 ■ Heel stick.

Rationale: Friction produces local heat, which aids vasodilation.

3. Blot the site dry completely with a dry gauze square before lancing.

   Rationale: Alcohol is irritating to injured tissue and it may also produce hemolysis.

4. With a quick, piercing motion, puncture the lateral heel with a microlancet. Be careful not to puncture too deeply. Optimal penetration is 4 mm.

5. Wipe the first drop of blood away with the gauze.

   Rationale: The first drop may be contaminated by skin contact and the blood cells may have been traumatized during the stick. Blood glucose may be lowered by residual alcohol.

Collecting the Blood Sample

1. Use transfer pipette to place a drop of blood on the glucose reflectance meter.

2. Use the capillary tube for hematocrit testing.

Prevent Excessive Bleeding

1. Apply a folded gauze square to the puncture site and secure it firmly with a bandage.
2. Check the puncture site frequently for the first hour after sampling.

Documentation

Record the findings and interventions taken on the infant's chart. Document the confirmatory laboratory-determined glucose level if hypoglycemia is suspected.

PERFORMING AN INTRAPARTAL VAGINAL EXAMINATION

Preparation

1. Explain the procedure, the indications for the exam, what the exam may feel like, and that it may cause discomfort.
2. Assess for latex allergies.
3. Position the woman with her thighs flexed and abducted. Instruct her to put the heels of her feet together. Drape the woman with a sheet, leaving a flap to access the perineum.

   Rationale: This position provides access to the woman's perineum. The drape ensures privacy.

4. Encourage the woman to relax her muscles and legs.

   Rationale: Relaxation decreases muscle tension and increases comfort.

5. Inform the woman before touching her. Be gentle.

Equipment and Supplies

- Clean disposable gloves if membranes are not ruptured
- Sterile gloves if membranes are ruptured
- Lubricant
- Nitrazine test tape

- Slide
- Sterile cotton-tipped swab (Q-tip)

Before the Procedure: Test for Fluid Leakage

If fluid leakage has been reported or noted, use Nitrazine test tape and Q-tip with slide for fern test before performing the exam.

> **Rationale:** As long as lubricant has not been used, Nitrazine tape registers a change in pH if amniotic fluid is present.

Procedure (Sterile if membranes ruptured)

1. Pull glove onto dominant hand.

   Rationale: Single glove is worn when membranes are intact. If a sterile exam is needed, both hands will be gloved with sterile gloves.

2. Using your gloved hand, position the hand with the wrist straight and the elbow tilted downward. Insert your well-lubricated second and index fingers of the gloved hand gently into the vagina until they touch the cervix. Use care when positioning your hand.

   Rationale: This position allows the fingertips to point toward the umbilicus and find the cervix.

3. If the woman verbalizes discomfort, acknowledge it and apologize. Pause for a moment and allow her to relax before progressing.

   Rationale: This validates the woman's discomfort and helps her feel more in control.

4. To determine the status of labor progress, perform the vaginal examination during and between contractions.

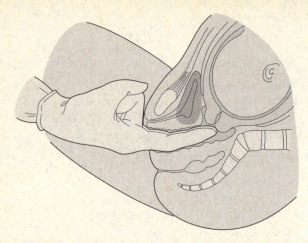

Figure 9 ▪ To gauge cervical dilatation, the nurse places the index and middle fingers against the cervix and determines the size of the opening. Before labor begins, the cervix is long (approximately 2.5 cm [1 in.]), the sides feel thick, and the cervical canal is closed, so an examining finger cannot be inserted. During labor, the cervix begins to dilate, and the size of the opening progresses from 1 cm to 10 cm (0.4 in. to 3.9 in.) in diameter.

> **Rationale:** Cervical effacement, dilatation, and fetal station are affected by the presence of a contraction.

5. Palpate for the opening, or a depression, in the cervix. Estimate the diameter of the depression to identify the amount of dilatation (see Figure 9).

> **Rationale:** Allows determination of effacement and dilatation.

6. Determine the status of the fetal membranes by observing for leakage of amniotic fluid. If fluid is expressed, test for amniotic fluid.

7. Palpate the presenting part (see Figure 10).

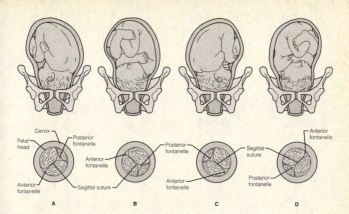

Figure 10 ■ Palpation of the presenting part (the portion of the fetus that enters the pelvis first). *A,* Left occiput anterior (LOA). The occiput (area over the occipital bone on the posterior part of the fetal head) is in the left anterior quadrant of the woman's pelvis. When the fetus is in LOA, the posterior fontanelle (located just above the occipital bone and triangular in shape) is in the upper left quadrant of the maternal pelvis. *B,* Left occiput posterior (LOP). The posterior fontanelle is in the lower left quadrant of the maternal pelvis. *C,* Right occiput anterior (ROA). The posterior fontanelle is in the upper right quadrant of the maternal pelvis. *D,* Right occiput posterior (ROP). The posterior fontanelle is in the lower right quadrant of the maternal pelvis.

Note: The anterior fontanelle is diamond shaped. Because of the roundness of the fetal head, only a portion of the anterior fontanelle can be seen in each of the views, so it appears to be triangular in shape.

Rationale: Determination of the presenting part is necessary to assess the position of the fetus and to evaluate fetal descent.

8. Assess the fetal descent (see Figure 11) and station by identifying the position of the posterior fontanelle.

9. Record findings on woman's chart and on fetal monitor strip if fetal monitor is being used.

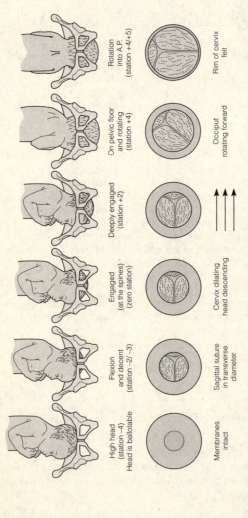

Figure 11 ■ Top: The fetal head progressing through the pelvis. Bottom: The changes that the nurse will detect on palpation of the occiput through the cervix while doing a vaginal examination.

Source: *Textbook for Midwives* (p. 246), by M. F. Myles, 1975, Edinburgh, Scotland: Churchill-Livingstone.

High head
(station -4)
Head is ballotable

Flexion
and decent
(station -2/ -3)

Engaged
(at the spines)
(zero station)

Deeply engaged
(station +2)

On pelvic floor
and rotating
(station +4)

Rotation
into A.P
(station +4/+5)

Membranes
intact

Sagittal suture
in transverse
diameter

Cervix dilating
head descending

Occiput
rotating forward

Rim of cervix
felt

PERFORMING GAVAGE FEEDING

Preparation

1. When choosing the catheter size, consider the size of the infant, the area of insertion (oral or nasal), and the desired rate of flow.

   Rationale: The size of the catheter will influence the rate of flow.

   Rationale: The very small infant (less than 1,600 g) requires a #5 Fr. feeding tube; an infant greater than 1,600 g may tolerate a larger tube. The size of the catheter will also influence the rate of flow.

2. Explain the procedure to the parents.
3. Elevate the head of the bed and position the infant on the back or side to allow easy passage of the tube.
4. Measure the distance from the tip of the ear to the nose to the xiphoid process, and mark the point with a small piece of paper tape (Figure 12) to ensure enough tubing to enter the stomach.

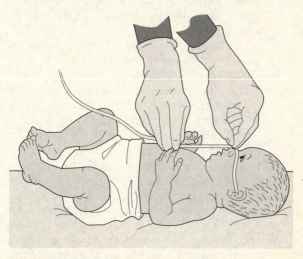

Figure 12 ■ Measuring gavage tube length.

Equipment and Supplies

- No. 5 or no. 8 Fr. feeding tube
- 3- to 5-mL syringe, for aspirating stomach contents
- 1/4-in. paper tape, to mark the tube for insertion depth and to secure the catheter during feeding
- Stethoscope, for auscultating the rush of air into the stomach when testing the tube placement
- Appropriate formula
- Small cup of sterile water to test for tube placement and to act as lubricant

> **Rationale:** Orogastric insertion is preferable to nasogastric because most infants are obligatory nose breathers. If nasogastric is used, a #5 Fr. catheter should be used to minimize airway obstruction.

Procedure: Clean Gloves
Inserting and Checking Placement of Tube

1. If inserting the tube nasally, lubricate the tip in a cup of sterile water. Use water instead of an oil-based lubricant, in case the tube is inadvertently passed into a lung. Shake any excess drops to prevent aspiration.

2. If inserting the tube orally, the oral secretions are enough to lubricate the tube adequately.

3. Stabilize the infant's head with one hand and pass the tube via the mouth (or nose) into the stomach to the point previously marked. If the infant begins coughing or choking or becomes cyanotic or phonic, remove the tube immediately, as the tube has probably entered the trachea.

4. If no respiratory distress is apparent, lightly tape the tube in position, draw up 0.5 to 1 mL of air into the syringe, and connect the syringe to the tubing. Place the stethoscope over the epigastrium and briskly inject the air (Figure 13). You will hear a sudden rush as the air enters the stomach.

5. Aspirate the stomach contents with the syringe, and note the amount, color, and consistency to evaluate

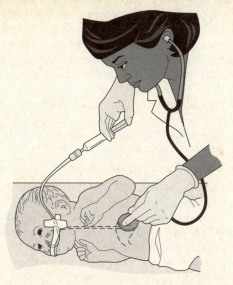

Figure 13 ▨ Auscultation for placement of gavage tube.

the infant's feeding tolerance. Return the residual to the stomach unless you are asked to discard it. It is usually not discarded because of the potential for electrolyte imbalance.

6. If the aspirated contents contain only a clear fluid or mucus and if it is unclear whether or not the tube is in the stomach, test the aspirate for pH. Stomach aspirate has a pH between 1 and 3.

Administering the Feeding

1. Hold the infant for feeding, or position the infant on the right side.

   Rationale: This position decreases the risk of aspiration in case of emesis during feeding.

2. Separate the syringe from the tube, remove the plunger from the barrel, reconnect the barrel to the tube, and pour the formula into the syringe.

3. Elevate the syringe 6 to 8 in. over the infant's head, and allow the formula to flow by gravity at a slow, even rate. You may need to initiate the flow of formula by inserting the plunger of the syringe into the barrel just until you see formula enter the feeding tube. Do not use pressure.

4. Regulate the rate to prevent sudden stomach distention leading to vomiting and aspiration. Continue adding formula to the syringe until the infant has absorbed the desired volume.

Clearing and Removing the Tube

1. Clear the tubing with 2 to 3 mL sterile water or with air.

2. To remove the tube, loosen the tape, fold the tube over on itself, and quickly withdraw the tube in one smooth motion to minimize the potential for fluid aspiration as the tube passes the epiglottis. If the tube is to be left in, position it so that the infant is unable to remove it. Replace the tube per hospital policy.

   Rationale: This ensures that the infant has received all of the formula. If the tube is going to be left in place, clearing it will decrease the risk of clogging and bacterial growth in the tube.

Maximize the Feeding Pleasure of the Infant

1. Whenever possible, hold the infant during gavage feeding. If it is too awkward to hold the infant during feeding, be sure to take time for holding after the feeding.

   Rationale: Feeding time is important to the infant's tactile sensory input.

2. Offer a pacifier to the infant during the feeding.

   Rationale: Sucking during feeding comforts and relaxes the infant, making the formula flow more easily. Infants can lose their sucking reflexes when fed by gavage for long periods.

PERFORMING LEOPOLD'S MANEUVERS

Leopold's maneuvers are a systematic way to evaluate the woman's abdomen to determine fetal position and presentation. Frequent practice increases the examiner's skill. Leopold's maneuvers may be difficult to perform on an obese woman or on a woman who has excessive amniotic fluid.

Preparation

1. Have the woman empty her bladder.

   Rationale: Palpating the abdomen may be uncomfortable if the woman's bladder is full. A full bladder may also make it difficult to complete the third and fourth maneuvers. See later discussion.

2. Ask the woman to lie on her back with her feet on the bed and her knees bent.

   Rationale: This position provides good access to the woman's abdomen. Flexing the knees helps relax the abdominal muscles.

3. Perform the procedure between contractions.

   Rationale: It is difficult to identify fetal parts when the abdominal muscles are contracted.

Procedure

1. First maneuver: Facing the woman, palpate the upper abdomen with both hands. Note the shape, consistency, and mobility of the palpated part (see Figure 14A).

   Rationale: The fetal head is firm, hard, and round and moves independently of the trunk. The breech (fetal buttocks) feels softer and symmetric and has small bony prominences; it moves with the trunk.

2. Second maneuver: After determining whether the head or buttocks occupies the fundus, try to determine the location of the fetal back. Still facing the woman, palpate the abdomen with gentle but deep pressure,

using the palms. Hold the right hand steady while the left hand explores the right side of the uterus. Then repeat the maneuver, holding the left hand steady while exploring the left side of the woman's abdomen with your right hand (see Figure 14B).

Rationale: The fetal back, on one side of the abdomen, feels firm and smooth and should connect what was found in the fundus with a mass in the outlet. The fetal extremities, which feel small and knobby, should be found on the other side.

3. Third maneuver: Determine what fetal part is lying just above the pelvic outlet. To do this, gently grasp the abdomen with the thumb and fingers just above the symphysis pubis. Note whether the presenting part feels like the fetal head or buttocks and whether it is engaged (see Figure 14C).

Rationale: This maneuver yields the opposite information from that gained with the first maneuver and validates the presenting part. If the head is presenting and is not engaged, it may be gently pushed back and forth.

4. Fourth maneuver: Facing the woman's feet, place both hands on the lower abdomen and move the hands gently down the sides of the uterus toward the pubis. Attempt to locate the cephalic prominence or brow (see Figure 14D).

Rationale: The brow is located on the side where there is the greatest resistance to the descent of the fingers toward the pubis. It is located on the side opposite the fetal back if the head is well flexed. However, when the fetal head is extended, the occiput is the first cephalic prominence felt, and it is located on the same side as the fetal back. Thus when completing the fourth maneuver, if the first cephalic prominence palpated is on the same side as the back, the head is not flexed. If the cephalic prominence is found opposite the back, the head is well flexed.

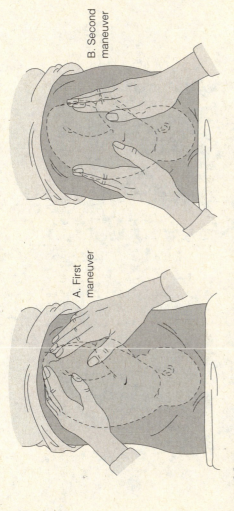

A. First maneuver

B. Second maneuver

Figure 14 ■ Leopold's maneuvers for determining fetal position, presentation, and lie.

Note: Many nurses do the fourth maneuver first to identify the part of the fetus in the pelvic inlet.

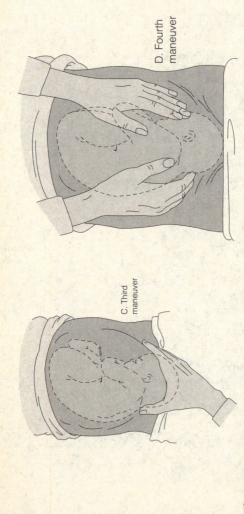

C. Third maneuver

D. Fourth maneuver

Figure 14 (continued) ■ Leopold's maneuvers for determining fetal position, presentation, and lie.

Note: Many nurses do the fourth maneuver first to identify the part of the fetus in the pelvic inlet.

PERFORMING NASAL PHARYNGEAL SUCTIONING

Preparation

1. Suction equipment is always available in the birthing area to clear secretions from the newborn's nose or oropharynx if respirations are depressed or if amniotic fluid was meconium stained.

2. Tighten the lid on the DeLee mucus trap or other suction device collection bottle.

   Rationale: This avoids spillage of secretions and prevents air from leaking out of the lid.

3. Connect one end of the DeLee tubing to low suction.

Equipment and Supplies

- DeLee mucus trap or other suction device

Procedure

1. Don gloves.

2. Without applying suction, insert the free end of the DeLee tubing 3 to 5 in. into the newborn's nose or mouth (Figure 15).

   Rationale: Applying suction while passing the tube would interfere with smooth passage of the tube.

3. Place your thumb over the suction control and begin to apply suction. Continue to suction as you slowly remove the tube, rotating it slightly.

   Rationale: Suctioning during withdrawal removes fluid and avoids redepositing secretions in the newborn's nasopharynx.

4. Continue to reinsert the tube and provide suction for as long as fluid is aspirated.

   Rationale: Excessive suctioning can cause vagal stimulation, which decreases the heart rate.

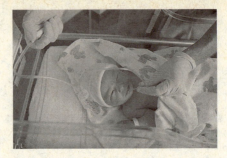

Figure 15 ■ DeLee mucous trap being used to suction a newborn's mouth to remove excess secretions.

5. If it is necessary to pass the tube into the newborn's stomach to remove meconium secretions that the newborn swallowed before birth, insert the tube through the newborn's mouth into the stomach. Apply suction and continue to suction as you withdraw the tube.

   Rationale: Because the newborn's nares are small and delicate, it is easier and faster to pass the suction tube through the mouth.

6. Document the completion of the procedure and the amount and type of secretions.

   Rationale: This documentation provides a record of the intervention and the status of the infant at birth.

POSTPARTUM PERINEAL ASSESSMENT

Preparation

1. Explain the purpose and the procedure for assessing the perineum during the postpartum period.

   Rationale: Typically, perineal assessment is the final step of the postpartum assessment.

2. Complete the assessment of fundal height and lochia as described in Clinical Skill: Assessing the Status of the Uterine Fundus after Birth and Clinical Skill: Evaluating Lochia.

3. At this point in a postpartal assessment, the woman is lying on her back with her knees flexed. Her perineal pad has already been lifted away from her perineum to permit inspection of the lochia. If an episiotomy was performed or if the birth was difficult, the woman may be using an ice pack on her perineum to reduce swelling. The ice pack would also have been removed for inspection of the lochia.

4. Ask her to turn onto her side with her upper knee drawn forward and resting on the bed (Sims' position).

   Rationale: When the woman is supine, even with her knees flexed, it is very difficult to expose the posterior portion of the perineum. Thus, the Sims' position makes it easiest to inspect the perineum and anal area.

Equipment and Supplies
- Clean perineal pad, clean ice pack if desired/needed
- Small light source such as a penlight may be necessary

Procedures: Clean Gloves
1. Use a systematic approach to assessment.

   Rationale: A systematic approach helps ensure that you don't overlook a significant finding.

2. In evaluating the perineum, begin by asking the woman's perceptions. How does she describe her discomfort? Does it seem excessive to her? Has it become worse since the birth? Does it seem more severe than you would expect?

   Rationale: Information from the client herself often helps identify developing problems.

Note: Pain that seems disproportionately severe may indicate that the woman is developing a vulvar hematoma.

3. After talking with the woman, assess the condition of the tissue. To allow for full visualization, it may

be helpful to ask the woman to lift the knee of her upper leg to expose her perineum more fully. In some cases it may help to use the nondominant hand to lift the buttocks and tissue. Note any swelling (edema) and bruising (ecchymosis).

Rationale: The tissue is often traumatized by the birth and mild bruising is not unusual. However, excessive bruising may indicate that a hematoma is developing.

4. Evaluate the episiotomy, if there is one, or any repaired laceration for its state of healing. Is it reddened? Note the edges of the incision. Are they well approximated? Tell the woman that you are going to palpate the incision gently, then do so. Note any areas of hardness. Note whether the incision is warmer to the touch than the surrounding tissue.

Rationale: Gentle palpation should elicit minimal tenderness and there should be no redness, warmth, or areas of hardness, which suggest infection. Both bruising and infection interfere with normal healing. Typically, within 24 hours the edges of the incision should be "glued" together (well approximated).

5. During the assessment be alert for odors. Typically the lochia has an earthy, but not unpleasant, smell that is easily identifiable.

Rationale: A foul odor associated with drainage often indicates infection.

6. Finally, assess for hemorrhoids. To visualize the anal area, lift the upper buttocks to fully expose the anal area (see Figure 16). If hemorrhoids are present, note the size, number, and pain or tenderness.

Rationale: Hemorrhoids often develop during pregnancy or labor and can cause considerable

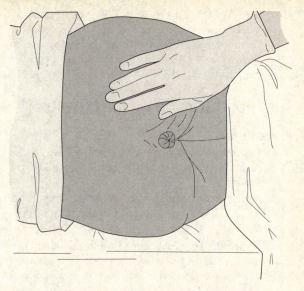

Figure 16 ■ Intact perineum with hemorrhoids.

discomfort. If hemorrhoids are present, the woman may benefit from available comfort measures.

7. During the assessment, talk to the woman about the effectiveness of comfort measures being used. Provide teaching about care of the episiotomy, hemorrhoids, and the like.

Rationale: Health teaching is an important part of nursing care. Many women have concerns about the episiotomy and may not know, for example, that the suture used is dissolvable. This is an excellent time to provide information about good health-care practices in both the short and long term.

8. Provide the woman with a clean perineal pad. Replenish the ice pack if necessary.

9. Record findings. For example: "Midline episiotomy; no edema, ecchymosis, tenderness, or discharge.

Skin edges well approximated. Woman reports pain relief measures are controlling discomfort." or "Perineal repair is approximated, minimal edema, no ecchymosis or tenderness; ice pack to perineum relieves pain."

THERMOREGULATION OF THE NEWBORN

Preparation

1. Prewarm the incubator or radiant warmer. Make sure warm towels and/or lightweight blankets are available.
2. Maintain the temperature of the birthing room at 22°C (71°F), with a relative humidity of 60% to 65%.

   Rationale: The change from a warm, moist intrauterine environment to a cool, dry, drafty environment stresses the newborn's immature thermoregulation system.

Equipment and Supplies

- Prewarmed towels or blankets
- Infant stocking cap
- Servocontrol probe
- Infant T-shirt and diaper
- Open crib

Procedure

1. Don gloves.

   Rationale: Gloves are worn whenever there is the possibility of contact with body fluids—in this case, a newborn wet with amniotic fluid, vernix, and maternal blood.

2. Place the newborn under the radiant warmer. Wipe the newborn free of blood, fluid, and excess vernix, especially from the head, using prewarmed towels.

Rationale: The radiant warmer creates a heat-gaining environment. Drying is important to prevent the loss of body heat through evaporation.

3. If the newborn is stable, wrap him or her in a pre-warmed blanket, apply a stocking cap, and carry the newborn to the mother. The mother and her support person can hold and enjoy the newborn together. Alternatively, carry the newborn wrapped to the mother, loosen the blanket, and place the infant skin-to-skin on the mother's chest under a warmed blanket.

Rationale: Use of a prewarmed blanket reduces convection heat loss and facilitates maternal-newborn contact without compromising the newborn's thermoregulation. Skin-to-skin contact with the mother or father helps maintain the newborn's temperature.

4. After the newborn has spent time with the parents, return him or her to the radiant warmer and apply a diaper. Leave the newborn uncovered (except for the cap and diaper) under the radiant warmer.

Rationale: Radiant heat warms the outer skin surface, so the skin needs to be exposed.

5. Tape a servocontrol probe on the newborn's anterior abdominal wall, with the metal side next to the skin. Do not place it over the ribs. Secure the probe with porous tape or a foil-covered aluminum heat deflector patch. Figure 17 shows a newborn with a skin probe. Note that in this picture the newborn is no longer wearing a stocking cap.

6. Turn the heater to servocontrol mode so that the abdominal skin is maintained at 36.4°C to 37.2°C (97.5°F to 99°F).

7. Monitor the newborn's axillary and skin probe temperatures per agency protocol.

Rationale: The temperature indicator on the radiant warmer continually displays the newborn's

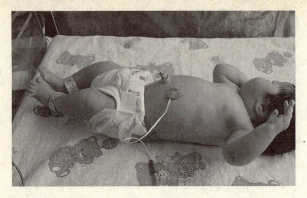

Figure 17 ■ Temperature monitoring for the newborn. A skin thermal sensor is placed on the newborn's abdomen, upper thigh, or arm and secured with porous tape or a foil-covered foam pad.

Source: Photographer, Elena Dorfman.

probe temperature. The axillary temperature is checked to ensure that the machine is accurately recording the newborn's temperature.

8. When the newborn's temperature reaches 37.2°C (99°F), add a T-shirt, double-wrap the infant (two blankets), and place the newborn in an open crib.

9. Recheck the newborn's temperature in 1 hour and regularly thereafter according to agency policy.

   Rationale: It is important to monitor the newborn's ability to maintain his or her own thermoregulation.

   Rapid heating can lead to hyperthermia, which is associated with apnea, increased insensible water loss, and increased metabolic rate.

10. If the newborn's temperature drops below 36.1°C (97°F), rewarm the infant gradually. Place the infant (unclothed except for a diaper) under the radiant warmer with a servocontrol probe on the anterior abdominal wall.

11. Recheck the newborn's temperature in 30 minutes, then hourly.
12. When the temperature reaches 37.2°C (99°F), dress the newborn, remove him or her from the radiant warmer, double-wrap, and place in an open crib. Check the temperature hourly until stable, then regularly according to agency policy.

Note: An infant who repeatedly requires rewarming should be observed for other signs and symptoms of illness and a physician should be notified, because the situation may warrant screening for infection.

APPENDICES

Appendices

APPENDIX A

COMMON ABBREVIATIONS IN MATERNAL-NEWBORN AND WOMEN'S HEALTH NURSING

AC	Abdominal circumference
accel	Acceleration of fetal heart rate
AFAFP	Amniotic fluid alpha-fetoprotein
AFI	Amniotic fluid index
AFP	Alpha-fetoprotein
AFV	Amniotic fluid volume
AGA	Average for gestational age
AI	Amnioinfusion
AMOL	Active management of labor
AOP	Apnea of prematurity *or* Anemia of prematurity
ARBOW	Artificial rupture of bag of waters
AROM	Artificial rupture of membranes
ART	Artificial reproductive technology
BAT	Brown adipose tissue (brown fat)
BBOW	Bulging bag of water
BBT	Basal body temperature
ß-hCG	Beta-human chorionic gonadotropin
BL	Baseline (fetal heart rate baseline)
BOW	Bag of waters
BPD	Biparietal diameter *or* Bronchopulmonary dysplasia
BPP	Biophysical profile
BRB	Bright red bleeding *or* Breakthrough bleeding
BR CA	Breast cancer
BSE	Breast self-examination
BSST	Breast self-stimulation test

CC	Chest circumference *or* Cord compression
CEI	Continuous epidural infusion
C–H	Crown-to-heel length
CID	Cytomegalic inclusion disease
CLD	Chronic lung disease
CM	Certified midwife
CMV	Cytomegalovirus
CNM	Certified nurse-midwife
CNP	Certified nurse practitioner
CNS	Clinical nurse specialist
CP	Chest pain
CPAP	Continuous positive airway pressure
CPD	Cephalopelvic disproportion *or* Citrate-phosphate-dextrose
CRL	Crown-rump length
CRNP	Certified registered nurse practitioner
C/S	Cesarean section (or C-section)
CST	Contraction stress test
CT	Chlamydia
CVA	Costovertebral angle
CVS	Chorionic villus sampling
D&C	Dilatation and curettage
D&E	Dilatation and evacuation
decels	Deceleration of fetal heart rate
DFMR	Daily fetal movement response
dil	Dilatation
DTR	Deep tendon reflexes
DV	Domestic violence
EAB	Elective abortion
ECMO	Extracorporeal membrane oxygenator
EDB	Estimated date of birth
EDC	Estimated date of confinement
EDD	Estimated date of delivery
EFM	Electronic fetal monitoring
EFW	Estimated fetal weight
EIA	Enzyme immunoassay
ELF	Elective low forceps
ELISA	Enzyme-linked immunosorbent assay
EP	Ectopic pregnancy
epis	Episiotomy
FAD	Fetal activity diary
FAS	Fetal alcohol syndrome
FASD	Fetal alcohol spectrum disorder

FBD	Fibrocystic breast disease
FBM	Fetal breathing movements
FBS	Fetal blood sample *or* Fasting blood sugar test
FCC	Family-centered care
FECG	Fetal electrocardiogram
FeSO$_4$	Iron supplement
FHR	Fetal heart rate
FHT	Fetal heart tones
Fhx	Family history
FL	Femur length
FMC	Fetal movement count
FMR	Fetal movement record
FPG	Fasting plasma glucose test
FSE	Fetal scalp electrode
FSH	Follicle-stimulating hormone
FSHRH	Follicle-stimulating hormone-releasing hormone
FSpO$_2$	Fetal arterial oxygen saturation
G or grav	Gravida
GC	Gonorrhea
GDM	Gestational diabetes mellitus
GIFT	Gamete intrafallopian transfer
GnRF	Gonadotropin-releasing factor
GnRH	Gonadotropin-releasing hormone
GTD	Gestational trophoblastic disease
GTPAL	Gravida, term, preterm, abortion, living children; a system of recording maternity history
HA	Head-abdominal ratio or headache
HAI	Hemagglutination-inhibition test
HC	Head compression
hCG	Human chorionic gonadotropin
hCS	Human chorionic somatomammotropin (same as hPL)
HIV	Human immunodeficiency virus
HMD	Hyaline membrane disease
hMG	Human menopausal gonadotropin
hPL	Human placental lactogen
HPV	Human papilloma virus
HRT	Hormone replacement therapy
HSV	Herpes simplex virus
ICSI	Intracytoplasmic sperm injection
IDM	Infant of a diabetic mother
IPG	Impedance phlebography

ISAM	Infant of a substance-abusing mother
IU	International units
IUD	Intrauterine device
IUFD	Intrauterine fetal death
IUGR	Intrauterine growth restriction
IUPC	Intrauterine pressure catheter
IUS	Intrauterine system
IVF	In vitro fertilization
LADA	Left-acromion-dorsal-anterior
LADP	Left-acromion-dorsal-posterior
LBC	Lamellar body count
LBW	Low birth weight
LDR	Labor, delivery, and recovery room
LGA	Large for gestational age
LH	Luteinizing hormone
LHRH	Luteinizing hormone-releasing hormone
LMA	Left-mentum-anterior
LML	Left mediolateral (episiotomy)
LMP	Last menstrual period *or* Left-mentum-posterior
LMT	Left-mentum-transverse
LOA	Left-occiput-anterior
LOF	Low outlet forceps
LOP	Left-occiput-posterior
LOS	Length of stay
LOT	Left-occiput-transverse
L/S	Lecithin/sphingomyelin ratio
LSA	Left-sacrum-anterior
LSP	Left-sacrum-posterior
LST	Left-sacrum-transverse
MAS	Meconium aspiration syndrome
mec	Meconium
mec st	Meconium stain
MLE	Midline episiotomy
MSAFP	Maternal serum alpha-fetoprotein
MUGB	4-methylumbelliferyl quanidinobenzoate
multip	Multipara
NEC	Necrotizing enterocolitis
NGU	Nongonococcal urethritis
NP	Nurse practitioner
NSCST	Nipple stimulation contraction stress test
NST	Nonstress test *or* Nonshivering thermogenesis
NSVD	Normal sterile vaginal delivery

NTD	Neural tube defects
NTE	Neutral thermal environment
OA	Occiput anterior
OC	Oral contraceptives
OCPs	Oral contraceptive pills
OCT	Oxytocin challenge test
OF	Occipitofrontal diameter of fetal head
OFC	Occipitofrontal circumference
OGTT	Oral glucose tolerance test
OM	Occipitomental (diameter)
OP	Occiput posterior
p	Para
Pap smear	Papanicolaou smear
PCA	Patient-controlled analgesia
PDA	Patent ductus arteriosus
PEEP	Positive end-expiratory pressure
PG	Phosphatidylglycerol *or* Prostaglandin
PID	Pelvic inflammatory disease
Pit	Pitocin
PKU	Phenylketonuria
PMS	Premenstrual syndrome
PNV	Prenatal vitamins
PPHN	Persistent pulmonary hypertension
Premie	Premature infant
primip	Primipara
PROM	Premature rupture of membranes
PSI	Prostaglandin synthesis inhibitor
PUBS	Percutaneous umbilical blood sampling
RADA	Right-acromion-dorsal-anterior
RADP	Right-acromion-dorsal-posterior
RDS	Respiratory distress syndrome
REM	Rapid eye movements
RIA	Radioimmunoassay
RLF	Retrolental fibroplasia
RMA	Right-mentum-anterior
RMP	Right-mentum-posterior
RMT	Right-mentum-transverse
ROA	Right-occiput-anterior
ROM	Rupture of membranes
ROP	Right-occiput-posterior *or* Retinopathy of prematurity
ROT	Right-occiput-transverse
RRA	Radioreceptor assay

RSA	Right-sacrum-anterior
RSP	Right-sacrum-posterior
RST	Right-sacrum-transverse
SAB	Spontaneous abortion
SET	Surrogate embryo transfer
SGA	Small for gestational age
SIDS	Sudden infant death syndrome
SMB	Submentobregmatic diameter
SOB	Suboccipitobregmatic diameter *or* Shortness of breath
SPA	Sperm penetration assay
SRBOW	Spontaneous rupture of bag of waters
SROM	Spontaneous rupture of membranes
STD	Sexually transmitted disease
STI	Sexually transmitted infection
STS	Serologic test for syphilis
SVE	Sterile vaginal exam
TAB	Therapeutic abortion
TC	Thoracic circumference
TCM	Transcutaneous monitoring
TDI or THI	Therapeutic donor insemination (*H* designates mate is donor)
TET	Tubal embryo transfer
TOL	Trail of labor
TORCH	Toxoplasmosis, rubella, cytomegalovirus, herpesvirus hominis type 2
TSS	Toxic shock syndrome
Ū	Umbilicus
UA	Uterine activity
UAC	Umbilical artery catheter
UAU	Uterine activity units
UC	Uterine contraction
UPI	Uteroplacental insufficiency
US	Ultrasound
VBAC	Vaginal birth after cesarean
VDRL	Venereal Disease Research Laboratories
VIP	Voluntary interruption of pregnancy
VLBW	Very low birth weight
VVC	Vulvovaginal *candidiasis*
WIC	Supplemental food program for Women, Infants, and Children
ZIFT	Zygote intrafallopian transfer

Appendix B
Conversions and Equivalents

Temperature Conversion

(Fahrenheit temperature − 32) × 5/9 = Centigrade temperature

(Centigrade temperature × 9/5) + 32 = Fahrenheit temperature

Selected Conversion to Metric Measures

Known Value	Multiply by	To Find
inches	2.54	Centimeters
ounces	28	Grams
pounds	454	Grams
pounds	0.45	kilogram

Selected Conversion from Metric Measures

Known Value	Multiply by	To Find
centimeters	0.4	inches
grams	0.035	ounces
grams	0.0022	pounds
kilograms	2.2	pounds

Conversion of Pounds and Ounces to Grams

Pounds	Ounces															
	0	1	2	3	4	5	6	7	8	9	10	11	12	13	14	15
0	—	28	57	85	113	142	170	198	227	255	283	312	340	369	397	425
1	454	482	510	539	567	595	624	652	680	709	737	765	794	822	850	879
2	907	936	964	992	1021	1049	1077	1106	1134	1162	1191	1219	1247	1276	1304	1332
3	1361	1389	1417	1446	1474	1503	1531	1559	1588	1616	1644	1673	1701	1729	1758	1786
4	1814	1843	1871	1899	1928	1956	1984	2013	2041	2070	2098	2126	2155	2183	2211	2240
5	2268	2296	2325	2353	2381	2410	2438	2466	2495	2523	2551	2580	2608	2637	2665	2693
6	2722	2750	2778	2807	2835	2863	2892	2920	2948	2977	3005	3033	3062	3090	3118	3147
7	3175	3203	3232	3260	3289	3317	3345	3374	3402	3430	3459	3487	3515	3544	3572	3600
8	3629	3657	3685	3714	3742	3770	3799	3827	3856	3884	3912	3941	3969	3997	4026	4054
9	4082	4111	4139	4167	4196	4224	4252	4281	4309	4337	4366	4394	4423	4451	4479	4508
10	4536	4564	4593	4621	4649	4678	4706	4734	4763	4791	4819	4848	4876	4904	4933	4961
11	4990	5018	5046	5075	5103	5131	5160	5188	5216	5245	5273	5301	5330	5358	5386	5415
12	5443	5471	5500	5528	5557	5585	5613	5642	5670	5698	5727	5755	5783	5812	5840	5868

(continued)

Conversion of Pounds and Ounces to Grams (continued)

	Ounces															
Pounds	0	1	2	3	4	5	6	7	8	9	10	11	12	13	14	15
13	5897	5925	5953	5982	6010	6038	6067	6095	6123	6152	6180	6209	6237	6265	6294	6322
14	6350	6379	6407	6435	6464	6492	6520	6549	6577	6605	6634	6662	6690	6719	6747	6776
15	6804	6832	6860	6889	6917	6945	6973	7002	7030	7059	7087	7115	7144	7172	7201	7228
16	7257	7286	7313	7342	7371	7399	7427	7456	7484	7512	7541	7569	7597	7626	7654	7682
17	7711	7739	7768	7796	7824	7853	7881	7909	7938	7966	7994	8023	8051	8079	8108	8136
18	8165	8192	8221	8249	8278	8306	8335	8363	8391	8420	8448	8476	8504	8533	8561	8590
19	8618	8646	8675	8703	8731	8760	8788	8816	8845	8873	8902	8930	8958	8987	9015	9043
20	9072	9100	9128	9157	9185	9213	9242	9270	9298	9327	9355	9383	9412	9440	9469	9497
21	9525	9554	9582	9610	9639	9667	9695	9724	9752	9780	9809	9837	9865	9894	9922	9950
22	9979	10007	10036	10064	10092	10120	10149	10177	10206	10234	10262	10291	10319	10347	10376	10404

Appendix C

Actions and Effects of Selected Drugs During Breastfeeding*

Anticoagulants

Coumarin derivatives (warfarin, dicumarol): Relatively safe to use; only small amount in breast milk; check PTT.

Heparin and derivatives (Lovenox): Does not cross into breast milk; check PTT.

Anticonvulsants

Phenytoin (Dilantin), phenobarbital: Generally considered safe; if high doses of phenobarbital are ingested, may cause drowsiness; short-acting phenobarbiturates (secobarbital) preferred, because they appear in lower concentration in milk.

Magnesium sulfate: Lactogenesis may be delayed.

---

*Based on data from Riordan, J. & Auerbach, K. J. (2005). *Breastfeeding and human lactation* (3rd ed., pp. 146–166). Boston: Jones & Bartlett; Briggs, G. G., Freeman, R. K., & Yaffe, S. J. (2008). *Drugs in pregnancy and lactation* (8th ed.). Baltimore: Williams & Wilkins; Hale, T. (2006). *Medications and mothers' milk* (12th ed.). Amarillo, TX: Pharmasoft Publishing; Committee on Drugs, American Academy of Pediatrics. (2001). The transfer of drugs and other chemicals into human milk. *Pediatrics, 108*(3), 776.

Antidepressants

SSRI class:

Fluoxetine (Prozac), fluvoxamine: Effect on newborn unknown but may be of concern.

Tricyclic antidepressants (doxepin): Sedation, potential respiratory arrest in infant.

Antihistamines

Diphenhydramine (Benadryl), Claritin, Allegra: May cause decreased milk supply; infant may become drowsy or irritable.

Clemastine (Tavist): Contraindicated.

Antihypertensives

β adrenergic blockers:

Atenolol, acebutolol: Cyanosis.

Tenormin: Hypotension, bradycardia.

Antimetabolites

Unknown, probably long-term anti-DNA effect on the infant; potentially very toxic.

Antimicrobials

Aminoglycosides: May cause ototoxicity or nephrotoxicity if given for more than 2 weeks.

Ampicillin: Skin rash, candidiasis; diarrhea.

Azithromycin: No risk to newborn.

Chloramphenicol (rarely used): Possible bone marrow suppression; too low a dose for Gray syndrome; refusal of breast.

Erythromycin: Accumulates in breast milk, idiopathic hypertrophic pyloric stenosis.

Methacycline: Possible inhibition of bone growth; may cause discoloration of the teeth; use should be avoided.

Metronidazole (Flagyl): Possible neurologic disorders or blood dyscrasias; delay breastfeeding for 12 hours after dose.

Penicillin: Possible allergic response; candidiasis.

Quinolones (synthetic antibiotics): Can cause arthropathies.

Sulfonamides: May cause hyperbilirubinemia; use contraindicated until infant is over 1 week old.

Tetracycline: Long-term use and large doses should be avoided; may cause tooth staining or inhibition of bone growth.

Antithyroids

Thiouracil: Contraindicated during lactation; may cause goiter or agranulocytosis.

Propylthiouracil: Safe; monitor infant thyroid function.

Barbiturates
Phenothiazines: May produce sedation.

Bronchodilators

Aminophylline: May cause insomnia or irritability in the infant.

Leukotriene inhibitors (Zyflo, Accolate): Potential tumorigenicity.

Caffeine

Excessive consumption may cause jitteriness or wakefulness.

Cardiovascular

Clonidine (Catapres): Reduces milk volume.

Methyldopa: Increases milk volume.

Propranolol (Inderal): May cause hypoglycemia; possibility of other blocking effects, especially if infant has renal or liver dysfunction.

Quinidine: May cause arrhythmias in infant.

Reserpine (Serpasil): Nasal stuffiness, lethargy, or diarrhea in infant.

Corticosteroids

Adrenal suppression may occur with long-term administration of doses greater than 20 mg/day.

Diuretics

Furosemide (Lasix): Not excreted in breast milk.

Thiazide diuretics (Esidrix, HydroDIURIL, Oretic): Safe but can cause dehydration, reduce milk production.

Heavy Metals

Gold: Potentially toxic; gold salts—compatible with breastfeeding.

Lead: Excreted in breast milk; high maternal levels can affect neuropsychologic development.

Mercury: Excreted in the milk and hazardous to infant.

Hormones

Androgens: Suppress lactation.

Thyroid hormones: May mask hypothyroidism.

Laxatives

Peri-Colace, Dulcolax: Relatively safe.

Milk of magnesia, Metamucil: Relatively safe.

Narcotic Analgesics

Codeine: Accumulation may lead to neonatal depression.

Meperidine: Avoid use. May lead to neonatal depression.

Morphine: Long-term use may cause newborn addiction.

Nonnarcotic Analgesics, NSAIDs

Acetaminophen (Tylenol): Relatively safe for short-term analgesia.

Ibuprofen (Motrin): Safe.

Propoxyphene (Darvon): May cause sleepiness and poor breastfeeding in infant.

Salicylates (aspirin): Safe after first week of life; monitor PTT.

Oral Contraceptives

Combined estrogen/progestin pills: Significantly decrease milk supply; may alter milk composition; may cause gynecomastia in male infants.

Progestin only (DMPA, Norplant): Safe if started after lactation is established.

Radioactive Materials for Testing

Gallium citrate (^{67}G): Insignificant amount excreted in breast milk; no breastfeeding for 2 weeks.

Iodine: Contraindicated; may affect infant's thyroid gland.

^{125}I: Discontinue breastfeeding for 24 hours.

^{131}I: Breastfeeding should be discontinued until excretion is no longer significant; may be resumed after 10 days.

Technetium-99m: Discontinue breastfeeding for 24 hours (half-life = 6 hours).

Sedatives/Tranquilizers

Diazepam (Valium): May accumulate to high levels; may increase neonatal jaundice; may cause lethargy, weight loss, and poor suck.

Lithium: Contraindicated; may cause neonatal flaccidity and hypotonia.

Smoking Cessation

Nicotine patch (Nicoderm, Nicotrol): Irritability, abnormal sleep patterns, poor feeding.

Bupropion (Zyban, Wellbutrin): No effect on breast-feeding.

Substance Abuse

Alcohol: Potential motor developmental delay; mild sedative effect.

Amphetamines: Controversial; may cause irritability, poor sleeping pattern.

Cocaine, crack: Extreme irritability, tachycardia, vomiting, apnea.

Marijuana: Drowsiness.

Heroin: Tremors, restlessness, vomiting, poor feeding.

Nicotine (smoking): Shock, vomiting, diarrhea, decreased milk production.

Appendix D
Selected Maternal Laboratory Values

Normal Maternal Laboratory Values		
Test	**Nonpregnant Values**	**Pregnant Values**
Hematocrit	37% to 47%	32% to 42%
Hemoglobin	12 to 16 g/dL**	10 to 14 g/dL**
Platelets	150,000 to 350,000/mm³	Significant increase 3 to 5 days after birth (predisposes to thrombosis)
Partial thrombo-plastin time (PTT)	12 to 14 seconds	Slight decrease in pregnancy and again in labor (placental site clotting)
Fibrinogen	250 mg/dL	400 mg/dL
Serum glucose		
Fasting	70 to 80 mg/dL	65 mg/dL
2-hour post-prandial	60 to 110 mg/dL	Less than 140 mg/dL
Total protein	6.7 to 8.3 g/dL	5.5 to 7.5 g/dL
White blood cell total	4500 to 10,000/mm³	5000 to 15,000/mm³
Polymorphonu-clear cells	54% to 62%	60% to 85%
Lymphocytes	38% to 46%	15% to 40%

**At sea level

Appendix E
Selected Newborn Laboratory Values

Normal Term Neonatal Cord Blood Laboratory Values

Test	Normal Values
Hematocrit	43% to 63%*
Hemoglobin	14 to 20 g/dL
Platelets	150,000 to 350,000/mm³
Reticulocyte	3% to 7%
White blood cell total	10,000 to 30,000/mm³
White blood cell differential	
Polymorphonuclear (segs)	40% to 80%
Lymphocytes	20% to 40%
Monocytes	3% to 10%
Serum glucose	45 to 96 mg/dL*
Serum electrolytes	
Sodium	126 to 166 mEq/L*
Potassium	5.6 to 12.0 mEq/L*
Chloride	98 to 121 mEq/L*
Carbon dioxide	13 to 29 mmol/L
Bicarbonate	18 to 23 mEq/L
Calcium	8.2 to 11.1 mg/dL
Total protein	4.8 to 7.3 g/dL

*All laboratory values are approximate. Consult your local laboratory for guidelines as to normal values.

Note: Adapted from Fanaroff, A. A., & Martin, R. J. (Eds.). (2006). *Neonatal-perinatal medicine* (8th ed.). Philadelphia, PA: Mosby.

APPENDIX F
SPANISH TRANSLATIONS OF ENGLISH PHRASES*

This appendix includes phrases you might find helpful in working with families during pregnancy, labor, and birth and after the birth. There are many ways to phrase questions. We have chosen some statements we consider essential and have tried to phrase them in a straightforward way. The phrases are designed to help you in situations in which translation is not possible at the moment.

This list begins with introductory statements, which are presented in a logical conversational flow. The remaining phrases are arranged according to the phases of pregnancy and birth during which they are most applicable.

Essential Introductory Phrases	Frases Introductoras Esenciales
Hello	Hola
I am a nurse.	Soy enfermera (enfermero).†
I am a student nurse.	Soy estudiante de enfermería.
My name is _____.	Mi nombre es _____.
	Me llamo _____.
What is your name?	¿Cuál es su nombre?
	¿Cómo se llama?
What name should I call you?	¿Cómo quiere que la llamemos?
	¿Cómo quiere ser llamada?

*Prepared by Elizabeth Medina, Ph.D. Associate Professor of Spanish, Regis University, Denver, Colorado.
†In Spanish, nouns that end in *a* indicate female gender; nouns that end in *o* indicate male gender.

Thank you	Gracias
Please	Por favor
Is someone here with you?	¿Hay alquien aquí con usted?
Does he (she) speak English?	¿Habla él (ella) inglés?
Goodbye	Adiós.

Phrases for the Antepartal Period	**Frases para el Periodo Prenatal**
Are you taking any medications now?	¿Está tomando algunas medicinas ahora?
Show me the medicine bottles please.	Por favor, muéstreme los frascos.
Have you ever had trouble with your blood pressure?	¿Ha tenido problemas alguna vez con la presión arterial?
When was the first day of your last period?	¿Cuál fue el primer día de su última regla? ¿Cuál fue el primer día de su última menstruación?
Have you had any spotting or bleeding since your last period?	¿Ha sangrado o ha tenido manchas de sangre desde su última regla?
Have you been on birth control pills?	¿Ha estado tomando píldoras anticonceptivas?
When did you stop taking them?	¿Cuándo dejó de tomarlas?
Do you have an intrauterine device (IUD)?	¿Usa un aparato intrauterino?
How many times have you been pregnant?	¿Cuántas veces ha estado usted embarazada?
Are you having any problems with your pregnancy?	¿Tiene problemas con su embarazo?
Is there anything that is worrying you?	¿Hay algo o alguna cosa que la preocupe?
I would like to take your blood pressure.	Quisiera tomarle la presió arterial.
I would like to take your pulse.	Quisiera tomarle el pulso.
I would like to take your temperature.	Quisiera tomarle la temperatura.

I would like to listen to your heart and lungs.	Quisiera escucharle el corazon y los pulmones.
I would like to check your uterus.	Quisiera examinarle el útero.
Please urinate in this cup and leave it in the bathroom.	Puede orinar en este vaso y dejarlo en el baño.
Please stand up.	Por favor, levántese.
Please sit down.	Por favor, siéntese.
Please lie down.	Por favor, acuéstese.

Phrases Related to Client Safety / **Frases Relacionadas con la Seguridad del Cliente**

I would like to talk to you alone.	Quisiera hablar a solas con usted.
Are you safe at home?	¿Sufre de peligros en casa?
Are you afraid of your partner?	¿Le tiene miedo a su compañero?
During your pregnancy has your partner hit, slapped, kicked, or punched you?	Durante su embarazo, ¿la ha golpeado? ¿la ha abofeteado? ¿la ha pateado? o ¿le ha dado puñetazos?
How many times?	¿Cuántas veces?
Do you have someone for support?	¿Cuénta con alguien que la pueda ayudar?

Questions the Mother or Father May Ask / **Posibles Preguntas que Madres o Padres Hacen**

How big is my baby?	¿De qué tamaño es el (la) bebé?
How much does the baby weigh now?	¿Cuánto pesa el bebé ahora?
When will I feel my baby move?	¿Cuándo lo (la) voy a sentir moverse?

Phrases for the Intrapartal Period / **Frases Durante el Parto**

Note: Review the essential introductory phrases for beginning a conversation.

Nota: Repase las frases introductoras para comenzar una conversación.

Are you having labor pains?	¿Tiene dolores de parto?
Are you having contractions?	¿Tiene contracciones?
Are you having pain?	¿Tiene dolores?
Do you need medicine for pain?	¿Necesita medicina para el dolor?
Do you need to urinate?	¿Necesita orinar?
This is a bedpan to urinate in.	Aquí tiene el bacín (la chata) (el pato) para orinar.
Can I help you to the bathroom?	¿La ayudo a ir al baño?
Do you need to have a bowel movement?	¿Necesita mover el vientre (obrar)? Necesita "Hacer caca"—coloquial
Has your bag of water broken?	¿Se le ha roto la bolsa de agua(s)?
Have you had any bright-red bleeding during your pregnancy?	¿Ha tenido algún sangramiento de color rojo durante su embarazo?
How many births have you had?	¿Cuántos niños le han nacido?
I need to do a vaginal examination.	Necesito hacerle un examen vaginal.
I will help you.	La voy a ayudar.
I will stay with you.	Me quedaré con usted.
Please pant. I will show you how.	Por favor, jadee. Le voy a mostrar cómo.
Do not push now.	No puje ahora.
Push now.	Puje ahora.
Stop pushing.	Pare de pujar. No puje más.
The doctor needs to do a cesarean birth.	El doctor le va a hacer una operación cesárea.
This is medicine for your pain. You will feel better soon.	Esta medicina es para el dolor. Va a sentirse mejor pronto.
When is your baby supposed to be born?	¿Cuando está supuesto a nacer el bebé?
January	enero
February	febrero
March	marzo
April	abril

May	mayo
June	junio
July	julio
August	agosto
September	septiembre
October	octubre
November	noviembre
December	diciembre
What is your doctor's name?	¿Cuál es el nombre de su doctor?
What is your midwife's name?	¿Cuál es el nombre de su comadrona (partera)?
Your baby is having some trouble now.	El bebé está pasando por algunos problemas. El bebé está sufriendo algunas dificultades.
I need to put this oxygen mask on you. It will help your baby. It may smell funny but it is OK.	Le voy a poner esta máscara de oxígeno. Va a ayudar al bebé. Huele extraño, pero no hay problemas.
Please turn on your left side.	Por favor voltéese al lado izquierdo.
Please turn on your right side.	Por favor voltéese al lado derecho.
Your baby is OK.	El bebé está bien.

Phrases for the Postpartal Period and the Newborn Area

Note: Review the essential introductory phrases for beginning a conversation.

Frases para el Periodo Despues del Parto y el Area del Recien Nacido

Nota: Repase las frases introductoras para comenzar una conversación.

Are you hungry?	¿Tiene hambre?
Are you thirsty?	¿Tiene sed?
Are you cold?	¿Tiene frío?
Are you tired?	¿Está cansada?
I am going to put antibiotic ointment in the baby's eyes.	Le voy a poner al bebé un ungüento antibiótico alrededor de los ojos.

It will help protect your baby from some infections.	Lo (la) va a proteger contra algunos infecciones.
I am going to take some blood from your baby's foot to check the blood sugar and hematocrit.	Le voy a sacar sangre del pie al bebé para determinar el azúcar de la sangre y el hematocrítico.
If your baby begins to spit up, please turn him (her) on his (her) side.	Si el bebé comienza a vomitar, colóquelo (colóquela) de costado.
It may help to position your baby like this.	Lo (la) ayudará—si lo coloca así. Lo (la) ayudaría—si lo colocara así.
I would like to suggest that you clean your nipples this way before you breast-feed your baby.	Es bueno que se lave los pezones de esta manera antes de darle el pecho al bebé.
It is better that you clean your baby's cord this way.	Es mejor para el bebé que le lave el ombligo de esta manera.
It is better that you bathe your baby this way.	Es mejor que lo (la) bañe de esta manera.
It is better that you clean your baby's penis this way.	Es mejor que le limpie el pene así.
I would like to suggest that you fold the diaper this way.	Le sugiero que doble el pañal así.
I would like to suggest that you fasten the diaper this way.	Le sugiero que asegure el pañal así.
Take the baby's temperature this way.	Tómele la temperatura así.
I need to check [your breasts, your uterus, your flow, your stitches, your legs and feet].	Necesito examinarle [los pechos, el útero, el flujo, los puntos, las piernas y los pies].
I need to feel your uterus.	Necesito examinarle el útero.
I need to massage your uterus.	Necesito darle un masaje en la región del útero.
Place your baby on its side.	Coloque al bebé de costado.
Place the baby's used diapers here.	Coloque aquí los pañales usados.
Please rub your uterus every half hour to keep it firm. I will show you how.	Necesita darse un masaje en la región del útero cada media hora para mantenerlo firme. Le voy a mostrar cómo.

Would you like to see your baby now?	¿Quiere ver a su bebé ahora?
Would you like me to help you feed your baby?	¿Quiere que le ayude a alimentarlo (la)?
Your baby needs a car seat to go home in.	El (la) bebé necesita un asiento para bebé en el automóvil.

Special Neonatal Needs
Necesidades del Recien Nacido

We are giving your baby oxygen.	Le vamos a dar oxígeno al (a la) bebé.
Your baby is having problems breathing.	El (la) bebé tiene problemas al respirar.
Your baby needs extra help.	El (la) bebé necesita ayuda especial.
Your baby needs to go to a special care nursery.	El (la) bebé necesita ir a la sala de cuidados especiales para bebés.

APPENDIX G

GUIDELINES FOR WORKING WITH DEAF CLIENTS AND INTERPRETERS

1. First, remember that it requires trust on the part of the client to allow nonsigning caregivers and an interpreter into her life.

2. It is important to use a registered interpreter. Medical interpreters are registered with the Registry of Interpreters for the Deaf. Although family members and friends may offer to interpret, it is best to use registered medical interpreters because they are required to translate the clients' and nurses' words accurately without adding in any other opinion.

3. Greet the client and family with a handshake and body posture that indicates welcome. You may point to your name tag and use the American Sign Language (ASL) alphabet cards to spell out your name. The client may wish to select cards to indicate her name. It is especially important as you work together to make the effort to provide a greeting as you would with speaking clients; greetings help develop rapport.

4. Once the interpreter is present, continue to look at the client and speak directly to her. There will be a

Prepared with the kind assistance of Mr. Gerald Dement, Interpreter Coordinator, Pikes Peak Center on Deafness, Colorado Springs, Colorado.

temptation to look at the interpreter, and it will help to remember that you are speaking to the client.

5. Avoid phrasing your words as if you are talking to the interpreter (e.g., "Can you tell her . . . ?"). Instead, phrase your questions as you do with speaking clients (e.g., "I'm going to ask you some questions now.").

6. Depend on the deaf client to ask questions.

7. Look at the client's face for signs of difficulty in understanding. Deaf clients have a behavior of "gesturing" that involves shaking their heads as if to indicate "yes" even when they do not understand. If the client is nodding "yes," ask her to repeat the directions you have just given.

8. Be as direct as possible. Keep to what you want to know or what you want to convey. Speak in short sentences, using nontechnical words. Avoid colloquial or slang words. Be sure to explain what you want to do before you do it. For instance, tell her you want to start an IV and explain the equipment. Then, with her permission, start the IV.

9. Be aware that deaf clients may have difficulty understanding when to take medications. It will be helpful to associate taking medications or completing some treatment or activity with meals. (For instance, while showing her the two capsules she is to take when she goes home, tell her to take the two capsules at breakfast and another two capsules at bedtime.) Avoid saying, "Take two capsules at 8:00 A.M., 2:00 P.M., and 12:00 A.M."

10. The difference in interpreting time may also affect obtaining a history. It is best to begin with a specific event in the past and work forward.

What to Do Until the Interpreter Arrives

1. Role-play as much as possible.

2. Demonstrate what you want the client to do or what you want to do.

3. Be resourceful.

4. Remember that some deaf clients can read lips. Some may read written language, but use care in assuming the client understands.

What to Do to Prepare for Working with a Deaf Client

1. Contact local agencies that work with deaf clients to see what resources are available. Ask about classes in ASL. Being able to use some basic signs will be very helpful while waiting for an interpreter to arrive.

2. Read to learn more about the deaf culture. Contact your local agency or the National Information Center on Deafness, Silver Springs, Maryland, to get suggestions on books you might read.

3. Investigate your health facility. What is available to assist you? Look for videos used for teaching in the maternal-child unit and note if they have captions. Remember that many deaf clients do not read written language, so it will be important to review the content of the video with an interpreter present.

Appendix H
Sign Language for Healthcare Professionals

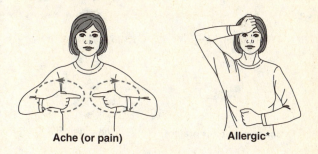

Ache (or pain)

Allergic*

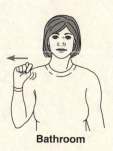

Bathroom

*Indicates signs that are in manually signed English. Those without an asterisk are in American Sign Language.

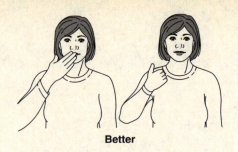

Better

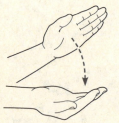
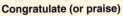

Congratulate (or praise)

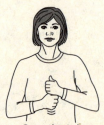
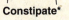

Constipate*

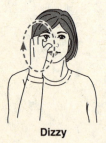

Dizzy

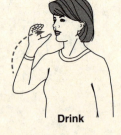

Drink

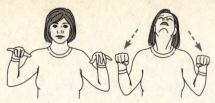

Faint

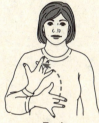

Feel

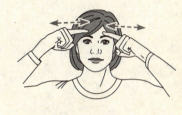

Headache

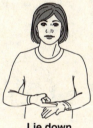

Lie down

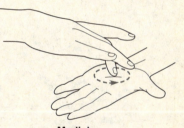

Medicine

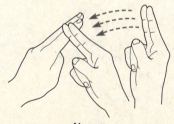

Name

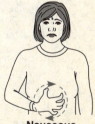

Nauseous

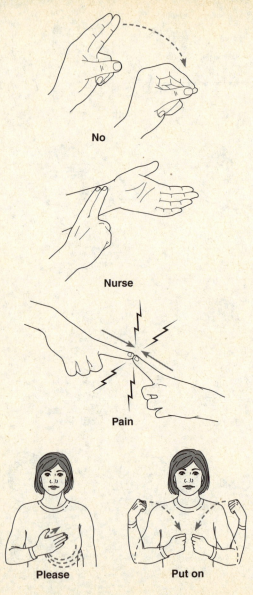

No

Nurse

Pain

Please

Put on

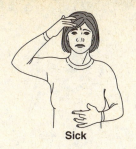

Sick

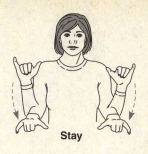

Stay

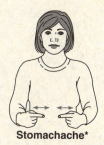

Stomachache*

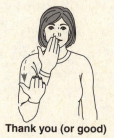

Thank you (or good)

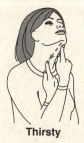

Thirsty

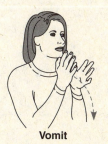

Vomit

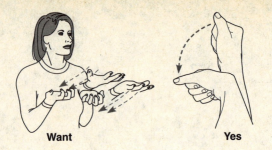

Want   Yes

INDEX

Note: Page numbers followed by *f* or *t* indicate figures and tables, respectively.

E

Ear(s), of newborns, physical assessment of, 161

Ear form and cartilage, of newborns, 152

Eclampsia. *See also* Preeclampsia-eclampsia
characteristics of, 43
management of, 46

Edema
ankle, pregnancy-related, relief from, 23
assessment for, during prenatal visits, 17

Effacement, cervical, assessment of, 79

Electronic fetal monitor, external, in FHR assessment, 81

Electronic fetal monitoring, 325–327. *See also* Fetal monitoring, electronic

Electronic uterine monitoring, external, during labor and birth, 77

Elimination
bowel, in postpartum assessment, 224*t*
in newborns, 165

Embolism
amniotic fluid, 124–126. *See also* Pulmonary embolism
pulmonary, 124–126. *See also* Pulmonary embolism

Emergency postcoital contraception, 249–250

Employment, during pregnancy, 25

Endometritis, 269

Engerix-B. *See* Hepatitis B vaccine

English phrases, Spanish translation of, 379–385

Episiotomy, postpartum discomfort due to, 217, 226

Epistaxis, pregnancy-related, relief from, 22

Epstein's pearls, in newborns, 162

Equivalents, conversions and, 368–370. *See also* Conversions and equivalents

Ergonovine, for subinvolution, 267

Erythromycin effects during breastfeeding, 372
for newborns, 156–157

Erythromycin ophthalmic ointment, 292–293
neonatal action of, 293
neonatal side effects of, 293
nursing considerations with, 294
pregnancy risk category for, 292
route, dosage, frequency of, 292

Estrogen/progestin in contraception, 246–248
effects during breastfeeding, 375

Exercise(s) in childbirth preparation, 26
postpartum, 232, 233*f*–234*f*
during pregnancy, 25–26

External electronic fetal monitor, in FHR assessment, 81

External electronic uterine monitoring, during labor and birth, 77

External version, 141–142
evaluation of, 142
nursing assessments during, 141
nursing diagnoses in, 141
nursing interventions during, 142

Extremity(ies)
lower, in postpartum assessment, 224*t*
of newborns, physical assessment of, 165

Eye(s), of newborns, physical assessment of, 161

Eyelid(s), of newborns, 161

F

Failure to progress, in labor, 109–112
evaluation of, 112
management of, 109–110
nursing assessments for, 110
nursing diagnoses in, 111
nursing interventions for, 111
sample nurse's charting in, 111–112

Faintness, pregnancy-related, relief from, 23

Family planning, 237–250. *See also* Contraception
barrier methods in, 239–244
contraceptive methods in, 237–250. *See also* Contraception
described, 237

G

Gallium citrate, effects during breastfeeding, 375

Gastrointestinal system, during pregnancy, 4

Gavage feeding, performing of, 343–347, 344f, 345f
clean gloves in, 344–347, 345f
equipment and supplies in, 343–344
preparation in, 343
procedure in, 344–347, 345f
administering feeding, 346
clearing and removing tube, 346–347
inserting and checking placement of tube, 344–346, 345f
maximizing feeding pleasure of infant, 346–347

GDM. *See* Gestational diabetes mellitus (GDM)

Genital(s) external, localized infection of, 269
female, 152
male, 152
of newborns, 152
physical assessment of, 163

Genital tract, lacerations of, management of, 262

Gestation, multiple, 67t–68t

Gestational age, problems related to, 114, 115t

Gestational age scoring, in newborns, 155–156, 156f

Gestational assessment, of newborns, 150, 151f

Gestational diabetes mellitus (GDM), 35–36

Gestational wheel, 15

Glove(s)
clean. *See* Clean gloves
sterile. *See* Sterile gloves

Glucose level, assessing of, in newborns, 157–158, 158f

Glucose monitoring, in diabetes mellitus, 37

Glucose screen, during prenatal visits, 17

Gold, effects during breastfeeding, 374

Gonorrhea
in newborns, 212
during pregnancy, 61t

Goodell's sign, 2

Grams, conversion of pounds and ounces to, 369–370

Grasp reflex, 166

Gravida, 8

Gravida/para notation, 8–9

Group B streptococcus, in newborns, 211–212

H

Hair, during pregnancy, 4

Head, of newborns, physical assessment of, 160, 161t

Health care providers for newborns, when to call, 171–172
sign language for, 389–394

Heart
in initial prenatal examination, 11
of newborns, physical assessment of, 162–163

Heart rate, fetal, auscultation of, 324–325. *See also* Fetal heart rate (FHR), auscultation of

Heartbeat, fetal, in due date determination, 15

Heartburn, pregnancy-related, relief from, 22

Heavy metals, effects during breastfeeding, 374

Heel stick, in newborn, 335–338, 336f, 337f
collecting blood sample in, 338
documentation of, 338
equipment and supplies in, 335–336
excess bleeding prevention in, 338
preparation in, 335, 336f
procedure in, 336–338, 337f

Heel to ear, in newborns, 154–155

Hegar's sign, 5

Hemabate. *See* Carboprost tromethamine (Hemabate)

Hematologic problems, of newborns, 188–196, 192f. *See also specific conditions, e.g.,* Anemia

Hematoma(s), management of, 262